W9-BYL-958

THE KETOGENIC DIET

A TREATMENT FOR EPILEPSY

THE

KETOGENIC

DIET

A

TREATMENT

FOR EPILEPSY

THIRD EDITION

Demos

Demos Medical Publishing, Inc., 386 Park Avenue South, New York, New York 10016

Library of Congress Cataloging-in-Publication Data

Freeman, John Mark.
  The ketogenic diet : treatment for epilepsy / John M. Freeman, Jennifer B. Freeman, Millicent T. Kelly.— 3rd ed.
        p.   cm.
  Previous editions published under title: The epilepsy diet treatment.
  Includes index.
  ISBN 1-888799-39-0 (pbk.)
  1. Epilepsy in children—Diet therapy. 2. Ketogenic diet. I. Freeman, Jennifer B. II. Kelly, Millicent T. III. Freeman, John Mark. Epilepsy diet treatment. IV. Title

RJ496.E6 F69 2000
618.92′8530654—dc21

                                                                    00-035856

Made in the United States of America

IMPORTANT NOTE TO READERS

This book will introduce the ketogenic diet to physicians, dietitians, and parents of children who might benefit from the treatment. It is not intended to be an instruction manual. It cannot take into account the specific needs of any individual patient. Like any course of treatment for epilepsy, a decision to try the ketogenic diet must be the result of a dialogue between parents and their child's physician. This diet should not be initiated except under the supervision of a physician and a trained dietitian or nurse. It should never be attempted by parents or patients alone.

OTHER TITLES BY JOHN M. FREEMAN, M.D.

Seizures and Epilepsy in Childhood: A Guide for Parents, Baltimore: Johns Hopkins University Press, 2nd Edition, 1997.

Tough Decisions: A Casebook in Medical Ethics, New York: Oxford University Press, 2nd Edition, 2000.

OTHER MATERIALS AVAILABLE ON THE KETOGENIC DIET

Videotapes:

- Introduction to the Ketogenic Diet: A Treatment for Pediatric Epilepsy (for the entire family)
- The Ketogenic Diet: A Treatment for Pediatric Epilepsy: A Kid's View
- The Ketogenic Diet: A Treatment for Pediatric Epilepsy: Doctor's Version

- A Primer in Calculating and Administering the Ketogenic Diet: A Dietitian and Nurse's Point of View

For copies of all videotapes, contact The Charlie Foundation to Help Cure Pediatric Epilepsy, 501 10th Street, Santa Monica, CA 90402.

KETO 2.0 COMPUTER PROGRAM: For copies, contact the Epilepsy Association of Maryland, 300 East Joppa Road, Suite 1103, Towson, MD 21204 (410) 828-7700. Computer disks are available to parents only on referral by a physician.

THE KETOGENIC COOKBOOK, by Dennis and Cynthia Blake, Penny-corner Press, Post Box 8, Gilman CT 06336, Phone (860) 873-3545, Fax (860) 873-1311, E-mail keto@pennycorner.com

Additional copies of this book may be obtained from Demos Medical Publishing, Inc., 386 Park Avenue South, New York, NY 10016, Phone: (800) 532-8663, Fax: (212) 683-0118, E-mail: orderdept@demospub.com

CONTENTS

SECTION IV: KETOGENIC COOKING

SECTION V: RECENT ADVANCES

SECTION VI: APPENDIXES

FOREWORD

On March 11, 1993, I was pushing my son, Charlie, in a swing when his head twitched and he threw his right arm in the air. The whole event was so subtle that I didn't even think to mention it to Nancy, my wife, until a couple of days later when it recurred. She said she had seen a similar incident. That was the beginning of an agony I am without words to describe.

Nine months later, after thousands of epileptic seizures, an incredible array of drugs, dozens of blood draws, eight hospitalizations, a mountain of EEGs, MRIs, CAT scans, and PET scans, one fruitless brain surgery, five pediatric neurologists in three cities, two homeopathists, one faith healer, and countless prayers, Charlie's seizures were unchecked, his development "delayed," and he had a prognosis of continued seizures and progressive retardation.

Then, in December 1993, we learned about the ketogenic diet and the success that Dr. John Freeman and Mrs. Kelly have been having with it at Johns Hopkins Hospital as a treatment for kids with difficult-to-control epilepsy. We took Charlie there, he started the diet. Charlie has been virtually seizure-free, completely drug-free, and a terrific little boy ever since. He has had to remain on a modified version of the ketogenic diet after being on the full diet for two years, but he goes to school and leads a normal, happy life. If we had had the information in this book 15 months earlier, a vast majority of Charlie's $100,000 of medical, surgical, and

drug treatment would not have been necessary, a vast majority of Charlie's seizures would not have occurred.

The publication of the first edition of *The Epilepsy Diet Treatment* was
supported by The Charlie Foundation so that other children and their
parents and doctors who struggle with this problem can be informed
about the ketogenic diet as perfected at Johns Hopkins. We hope this
book will help others decide whether the diet is a viable alternative to
their current treatment, and know that it will be a valuable guide once
the ketogenic diet has begun.

Jim Abrahams, Director
The Charlie Foundation to Help Cure Pediatric Epilepsy

PREFACE

"Yuck!" was once the common response to the ketogenic diet. It was the response of parents and, indeed, of many physicians who did not have experience with the diet. The very concept of a mere diet being able to control otherwise uncontrollable seizures seemed farfetched to many back in 1994, when we reintroduced the ketogenic diet with the initial publication of *The Epilepsy Diet Treatment: An Introduction to the Ketogenic Diet.*

Six years later, with the help of the first and second editions of *The Epilepsy Diet Treatment,* the ketogenic diet has once again become an accepted therapy for children with difficult-to-control seizures. It has won over skeptics and gained acceptance among both physicians and the public. A growing number of medical centers around the world are developing the expertise needed to administer the treatment successfully.

There is so much revised, updated, and new information, and the treatment is so well known now among those who might offer or benefit from it, that we decided to retitle this third edition as *The Ketogenic Diet: A Treatment for Epilepsy.*

What is new since the first edition of this book was published?

- New data from clinical studies and laboratory research have expanded our knowledge about many aspects of the ketogenic diet.

- Experience with hundreds of new patients has deepened our understanding of the best approaches to helping children and their families cope with the limitations and restrictions of the diet.

- Feedback and dialogue from many sources have been incorporated, ranging from neurologists to dietitians to comments from parents.

- New and improved menus have been added, including some developed by professional chefs whose children went through the diet.

- Instructions for calculating and managing the diet on a day to day basis have been revised to reflect the needs of modern dietitians.

- Ongoing laboratory research points toward potential future improvements in ketone measuring techniques, and searches to understand reasons for the diet's effectiveness.

The debate now taking place is not whether the diet is useful, but what place the diet should hold in the management of difficult-to-control seizures in children. Should it be offered after a child has failed all available medications? After she has failed two medications? Should it be limited to children over one year of age? Will it work in adults? (While we know of no reason why an adult should not attempt the diet, its efficacy and side effects in adults have not been widely studied.)

Even today, with all the new anticonvulsant medications that come on the market, there are still many children with difficult-to-control seizures. The ketogenic diet, though difficult, if properly done remains more effective than any of these new anticonvulsant medications. It seems clear that, if the diet were a drug, companies would be promoting it as the treatment of choice for difficult-to-control epilepsy.

The ketogenic diet should only be used under close medical supervision. The decision to use it should be the result of a dialogue between physicians and parents. It is rarely successful without the continuing support of an experienced physician and a knowledgeable dietitian.

The ketogenic diet is NOT the answer for everyone. But for some, it may result in a better quality of life with fewer side effects than any other therapy.

There remain many, many questions to be answered about the ketogenic diet. However, this new edition of *The Ketogenic Diet* reflects the many advances in understanding that have taken place since the book was first published six years ago.

John M. Freeman, M.D.

DEDICATION

Many happy stories have resulted from Charlie Abraham's success on the ketogenic diet. With the help of Jim and Nancy Abrahams, the Charlie Foundation created videotapes to introduce parents, children, doctors and dietitians to the diet. With the help of the Charlie Foundation, the first edition of this book was published. With the help of the Charlie Foundation, we have been able to train more than 27 medical centers to offer the ketogenic diet. With the support of the Abrahams family and the Charlie Foundation we have been able to start the diet in more than 350 children at Johns Hopkins since 1994, and to collect and analyze information crucial to the future understanding and acceptance of the diet.

For all of these accomplishments, and for the happy fact that the ketogenic diet has come back as an accepted, alternative form of antiepileptic therapy, we are deeply grateful for the dedication and support of Jim and Nancy Abrahams and of the Charlie Foundation. Few individuals have had as much impact on so many children in so short a time. None have changed the thinking of the medical community more quickly. We therefore rededicate this book to Jim and Nancy Abrahams on behalf of the many children who have been given new lives through the use of the ketogenic diet.

ACKNOWLEDGMENTS

We would like to acknowledge the parents and children who have been treated at Johns Hopkins and have so willingly cooperated with our ongoing clinical research by collecting information, returning for followup, and giving blood. The data we have accumulated was only partially supported by research grants. Without your help, we could not have accumulated the knowledge about the diet and its effects which has begun to convert skeptics into believers.

To the many physicians who have referred patients to the Johns Hopkins program and who have participated with and cooperated with our studies we express deep appreciation.

We also want to acknowledge those parents whose phone calls have been met with busy signals, or who have been placed on hold for long periods of time, and those who have had to wait for days to have their questions answered. To all of you, we send our apologies and hope for your understanding.

Within weeks after a TV program about Charlie Abrahams and the ketogenic diet aired on "Dateline" in 1994, the small staff of the Johns Hopkins Pediatric Epilepsy Center responded to more than 5,000 inquiries. The innumerable continued phone contacts from those parents who have brought their children to Johns Hopkins, and from those who are just interested in the diet, would have tried the patience of a less dedicated team. The close personal attention which has made the diet more acceptable to and more effective and manageable for many children could not have been accomplished without the staff's enduring talent and dedication.

We would specifically like to acknowledge and thank:

DR. EILEEN P.G. (PATTI) VINING, long time colleague and partner in this and many other endeavors to help children and families with epilepsy.

DIANA J. PILLAS, manager and coordinator-counselor of the Pediatric Epilepsy Center, whose tireless, indefatigable care and concern for parents and children with seizures or epilepsy has touched and improved untold numbers of lives.

JANE C. CASEY, RN, LCSWC, the Epilepsy Center's nurse clinician and dietitian-counselor, whose ability to manage children on the diet through sickness and health, and to assist the parents through good times and bad, has made their lives easier and better.

PAULA L. PYZIK, who has collected, coded, and analyzed the information about children on the ketogenic diet and who has made it possible to finally provide data, not merely impressions, about many clinical facets of the diet.

JANE MCGROGAN, RD, our dietitian now that Millicent Kelly has once again retired. Her dedication to helping the parents to "get it right" has assured the best nutrition and best chance at seizure control for all children embarking on the diet.

We must, of course, acknowledge our gratitude to the Epilepsy Center's secretaries past and present, who have done a yeoman's job juggling phone calls from parents who think their questions require an immediate answer and those whose calls have not yet been returned, while making appointments for children who wanted to see us yesterday.

Our thanks to Baltimore-based ketocoaches Gina and Gretchen Homer, who have visited almost every family during the admission process to provide encouragement and a sense of humor. And our thanks to the many parents who have served as ketocoaches all around the country to parents who are just starting on the diet. The support of those who have succeeded with the diet is invaluable to those facing the obstacles for the first time.

We also express our appreciation to the Almeida Family for their continuing contributions to the Alex Almeida Fund, which has been used to help families in need who are initiating the diet.

Lastly, all of this would not have come about without the commitment and dedication of Millicent T. Kelly, who has recently retired as the dietitian of the Epilepsy Center. It was through Millie that the wisdom of the diet was preserved through its years in the wilderness, and it was her dedication that helped to revive interest in the diet and to document its ability to improve the lives of many children. In the first edition of this book Millie added the quotation:

What I spent is gone
What I kept is lost
But what I gave away
Will be mine forever.

(Author unknown)

Millie is rich, indeed.

John M. Freeman

SECTION I

OVERVIEW

CHAPTER ONE

INTRODUCTION
TO THE
KETOGENIC DIET

Every child and every family who embarks on the ketogenic diet dreams of a total cure. Sometimes their dream comes true. Megan, a highly motivated 12-year-old with a supportive family, was able to "cure" her seizures after two years on the diet. Here is a letter written by Megan's parents after she had been on the diet for just six weeks.

MEGAN'S STORY

DEAR DR. FREEMAN,

I want to share with you and your team the wonderful changes in Megan's life since she has been on the ketogenic diet.

As you remember, we were having very serious and frightening prospects as a family. . . . Megan's seizures, which we called "stares," were out of control in spite of using three drugs. She was experiencing so many an hour that she was regressing both in school and in her personal skills. She would be unable to remember what she had been doing prior to a "stare," and therefore had difficulty staying focused on tasks— whether keeping her place in her reader or even dressing herself, or just remembering what she went to get in another room. . . . Being only 10 years old, she was very frightened because she was not able to stop "staring," and children teased her. She cried because she would wake up at night and not realize she was in her own bedroom. She also described many auras in which she reported seeing flashing lights and people's faces changing colors. . . .

We could not increase the Depakote level because of the side effects to her stomach. She was taking Mylanta three times daily just to coat her stomach to tolerate the Depakote. And still her stomach hurt, resulting in poor appetite—which . . . had reduced her weight to the tenth percentile for her age group. This constant concern over her eating patterns and small consumption had also created tension in our family over meals.

The . . . seizures also resulted in her . . . sleeping at least 12 to 13 hours out of each 24, including sleeping an hour at school midday.

As a result of all these physical changes, the disorder now took Megan's social life. Since she had to go to bed so early, she couldn't go to church or . . . school functions. On Saturdays, she could play only in the morning because she would sleep in the afternoon. Spending the night with a friend became out of the question because she didn't get enough sleep—which increased the "stares." Her neurologist recommended Johns Hopkins Hospital and your team because he felt surgery would have to be considered—that Megan would likely become worse . . . . And so we came, expecting to have to chance even losing her life in order to give her the chance of improving quality of life—and save the very essence of our spirited, enthusiastic, loving child.

Due to the complexity of Megan's neurological situation, you did not recommend surgery, but offered her something incredible—a diet! You told Megan she could use her strength to turn down sugar from her friends and to stay on her diet. We will never forget how her little face lit up when you said "no surgery."

Her life has literally turned around from that day. . . . She has been very dedicated to learning about labels with sugar, preparing foods, etc., and is determined to stay on her diet.

It has been and will be worth the extra time it requires to plan and prepare the meal plans. She has had only two "stares"—one the day of dismissal from the hospital, the other at school when she began decreasing the Dilantin level.

She has really had a learning spurt. Her reading teacher . . . tested Megan and . . . confirmed the improvement in reading already! Megan is thrilled to be promoted to a harder reader. Her memory also improved, and she is being assigned more difficult words. She is choosing her clothes and dressing herself with little supervision from me. She is going to slumber parties!

Family and friends say over and over they can tell how well she is doing. Her thoughts are well connected in conversation. Megan says, "I'm so much better than before I went to Baltimore. I can remember things now. I'm doing great!" In short, she is alert and happy.

After seven and a half years of dealing with frequent and frustrating medication changes with varying side effects, this diet is a fantastic alternative. I will not complain! This Christmas was our most joyous since the first Christmas after she was born. —MH

The diet was not easy. Megan's family had to learn step by step how to organize life around the diet for two whole years. Megan cried the time she won a spelling bee in her class and the prize was a pizza, of which she could take not even a single bite. "I shared it with all of the class, but I couldn't have any myself," she later recalled. Megan's own motivation, as well as her supportive family, were keys to making the diet a success. The fact that the diet was 100 percent successful was highly motivating and its own reward.

Megan remained on the diet for two years and has now been off the diet for eight years—seizure-free and medicine-free. Despite structural damage to her brain from the epilepsy and a mild hemiparesis, she has just graduated from high school and plans to go on to more studies. Asked if the diet was worth it, Megan replied, "It gave me my life back."

Megan's story is dramatic, but many similar letters have been written by grateful parents. Articles about children with 100 percent success stories have appeared in newspapers and periodicals around the country, with headlines such as "Michael's Magical Diet," "Cured by Butter,

Mayo and Cream," and "High Fat and Seizure Free." These are the glowing reports of the dramatic success that the diet can achieve.

Defining Success

Unfortunately, the ketogenic diet does not result in a success story for everyone. Almost half of all children who start the diet stop during the first year. Some stop because, despite the medical and support team's best efforts to "fine-tune" the diet (see Chapter 5), and despite the family's diligent efforts, the seizures have not improved sufficiently to make their efforts worthwhile. Some discontinue because of illness, noncompliance, or because the diet is "just too hard."

For example, Jay[1] was a 15-year-old whose seizures started at age 9 years. In 6th grade he had so many dizzy spells and seizures that he missed 77 days of school. In 7th grade he was taking 16 pills per day and still missed 108 days of school. He had brain surgery in which his temporal lobe was resected, but the seizures returned. Jay and his family then decided to try the ketogenic diet.

Jay's goal, like that of many teenagers, was to be able to drive. For this he needed to be 100 percent seizure-free. On the ketogenic diet he fell short of this goal—he was nearly seizure-free, but not completely. Five months after starting the diet, Jay's mother reported that he "lives on sausages, eggs and choked-down heavy cream at every meal." "We are always in the kitchen . . . cutting, cleaning, weighing," his parents wrote. "We never go out to eat anymore or have pizza at home. . . . At Thanksgiving the whole family ate eggs."

Jay's seizures were much improved and his medications were reduced, but without being seizure-free, Jay believed that he would never be able to drive and therefore the diet was too much trouble. The diet was discontinued after about nine months.

With so much improvement in seizure control, was Jay's experience with the diet a success? Well, yes and no. His seizures were markedly

---

[1]Some names in this book have been changed to protect the privacy of the patients.

decreased and his medications were reduced. However, his major reason for undertaking the diet was to become 100 percent seizure-free so that he could drive. Since he wasn't able to reach this goal, the diet was—for him—a failure.

Perhaps with current knowledge Jay's diet could have been fine-tuned to further improve seizure control. A more supportive and creative family might have found ways to go out for meals and spend less time in the kitchen, to make life on the ketogenic diet closer to normal. But Jay's family could not or did not. From the perspective of his support team at Johns Hopkins, Jay's experience with the diet was a failure not because it didn't completely eliminate his seizures, but because we thought (in our optimistic fashion) that it could have been a success but for variables beyond our control. Ultimately, however, it is the child and the parents who must define the diet's "success" or "failure."

WHO IS A CANDIDATE FOR THE KETOGENIC DIET?

We do not know who is the ideal candidate for the diet, nor do we know who, if anyone, should be refused the diet. The diet is equally effective throughout infancy, childhood, and early adolescence. It is effective in varied seizure types and with a widely different frequency of seizures. Without data we are convinced that the diet should *not* be reserved only for children who have failed all possible medications. Similarly, it should *not* be used merely because a child's parents "don't find medications natural."

The ketogenic diet is *not* the treatment of choice for people who have experienced only one seizure, or even for those who have had only a few seizures. If seizures can be successfully controlled by medication, then most will find that the rigors and sacrifices required by the diet are not worthwhile.

On the other hand, the ketogenic diet *should* be tried earlier in the child whose myoclonic-akinetic seizures are difficult to control with medications, and perhaps in the child with Lennox-Gastaut syndrome. The diet is less likely to work in the presence of a structural lesion, but still can be given a try before surgery. Its role in the treatment of infantile spasms is not known.

Sylvia is a good example of our uncertainty about who is a good candidate for the ketogenic diet. Brought to us when she was 18 months old, Sylvia had suffered constant seizures, despite good trials of medications, ever since she had experienced a very near sudden infant death syndrome (SIDS) episode at three months of age. The infant did not see, hear, or respond. She had not even cried for more than a year. Her mother asked us to try the ketogenic diet.

When asked what she hoped the diet would accomplish, Sylvia's mother replied that the baby would be easier to care for if the seizures were under better control. This seemed reasonable, so Sylvia was admitted for the diet. After fasting and two days of ketogenic formula, Sylvia started to cry. Her mom burst into tears of joy at the sound.

On the fifth day of the diet, Sylvia smiled. Her seizures decreased markedly, but did not come under control for almost nine months. After a year and a half on the diet, Sylvia was sitting and playing. She is now standing and interacting—drug-free and seizure-free. She remains severely mentally and physically impaired, but there *was* a little girl in there.

When considering who would be a good candidate for the diet, it is useful to keep in mind:

- 70 percent of people who have a single seizure will never have another.

- 70 percent of those who have a second seizure will have their seizures successfully controlled by medication.

- The ketogenic diet begins to be an option worth considering when two or more medications fail to bring about seizure control, or when medications cause unacceptable side effects.

- If a first medication fails, the chance that a second or third will also be ineffective rises.

- For approximately one-fifth (20 percent) of children with epilepsy, even the newer medications are either ineffective in controlling seizures or have unacceptable side effects. There is little evidence, but much hope, that the next new medication will provide better seizure control.

Even with seizures under fairly good under control, medication may affect children's alertness and mental clarity, impairing their ability to learn and reach their full potential. Therapy for epilepsy is often a balance between seizure control and medication toxicity.

The point at which an individual's seizures are deemed out of control, or side effects are considered unacceptable, varies from person to person and from family to family. One hundred seizures a day is clearly too many, but are three seizures a month too many? Some children and families consider limiting seizures to one a week a victory, while others consider one seizure every two months an intolerable state of affairs. Varying degrees of sedation, hyperactivity, and learning disabilities may be acceptable in exchange for seizure control. But what if you could control seizures without such side effects?

This is a question asked by many parents. Could my child learn better, faster, more easily without the toxicity of the medication? Would her behavior and attention improve if she weren't on anticonvulsants? How can you tell when a child cannot be taken off medication without the chance of recurrent seizures?

The net result is that many children and their parents look beyond currently available medications for a satisfying solution to seizure treatment. For many parents, the ketogenic diet, which does not have the cognitive and behavioral side effects of anticonvulsant medications, offers a chance—sometimes an unattainable dream—of seeing their child free of medications and seizures. For many parents, it is as important to see their child free of medication as to see them free of seizures. For others, like the family of "Jay" described previously, the ketogenic diet is not considered a success because the seizures were not completely eliminated. Even in those who discontinue the diet, however, most find the attempt at the diet worthwhile because, as they often say, "at least we know that we tried."

The ketogenic diet is a rigid, mathematically calculated, doctor-supervised therapy. It is high in fat and low in carbohydrate and protein, containing three to five times as much fat as carbohydrate and protein combined. Calories and

liquid intake are strictly limited. This diet should not be attempted except under close supervision by a physician.

MICHAEL IS DRUG-FREE AND SEIZURE-FREE! He was singing "Jingle Bells" last week, but changed the words to something like this:

> *Jingle Bells, I'm a special kid,*
> *'Cause I'm on the magic diet.*
> *Oh, what fun it's gonna be*
> *To not have seizures anymore!*

Isn't that something? We laughed so hard, we cried. Like so many Americans, my faith lay in drugs or surgery. . . . My feelings now cannot be adequately expressed. The meals do take time to prepare, and there are other difficult things to get through, but it's working! IT'S WORKING! Michael is a different child being off the drugs. More alert, more physical, more talkative (boy, is he!). More everything. I feel we now have a whole child. All because of a diet. I would not wish this diet on my worst enemy, but I would wish it on every child with uncontrolled seizures. It could be the beginning of a whole new life. —EH

The ketogenic diet improves control of seizures in more than half of the children who try it. Only 10 percent of children with very difficult-to-control seizures have their seizures completely controlled, but one-third have their seizures mostly controlled, most have medication reduced, and some become free of medication.

Burning fat

The human body has been designed and modified over time to meet potential emergency conditions. Thus, the normal person has stores of energy in reserve (glucose and glycogen) to use when food is not immediately available. If no new sources of glucose are available within 24 to 36 hours, these stores are used up and the body begins to burn energy that it has stored as fat.

Fasting has been recognized as a means of controlling seizures since biblical times. But fasting as a treatment for seizures has one major drawback, namely, people cannot fast indefinitely because they would starve to death! The body would run out of fat and then burn its own muscle (protein). Even if seizures were controlled by fasting, they often would return when a normal diet was resumed. However, in the early 1900s fasting for 10 or even 20 days was used as a treatment for seizures and formed the basis for the development of the ketogenic diet.

The ketogenic diet simulates the metabolism of a fasting body. A fasting person burns stored body fat for energy; a person on the ketogenic diet derives energy principally by burning the fat in the diet rather than from the more common energy source, carbohydrate (glucose). As the water content of a fasting body is lower than normal, so the ketogenic diet limits liquid intake and lowers the water content of the body. But unlike fasting, the ketogenic diet allows a person to maintain this fat-burning, partially dehydrated metabolism over an extended period of time.

I CALL IT THE "VOODOO DIET." My son remembers when he was on the medication. He calls it "when I was bad" or "when I couldn't control myself." He used to rock back and forth, flip the light switch fifty times, make loud noises, bite himself, bite other people, put his hand in a flame, you name it. His seizures were fairly well controlled; he was only having maybe one a month or every six weeks. His doctor said, "This kid's seizures are pretty much under control on the medicine. What more do you want?" What I wanted was for my boy to get his old, sweet personality back.

He has had no seizures or medication for a year and a half on the diet. He likes himself now. He is content with who he is. I can hardly believe it. Anyone who sees him can hardly believe he is the same kid. I am certainly glad that I tried this diet, despite the fact that it ties you to the house and it ties you to the meals. I hate the diet. I mean, the minute it's over I'm going to bomb my food scale. But it has helped my son so immensely that I can't hate it too much. —CC

SAMPLE MEAL PLANS

The ketogenic diet presented in this book is based on the protocol devised by Dr. Samuel Livingston, who was director of the Pediatric Seizure Clinic at the Johns Hopkins Hospital from 1934 to 1971. The most substantial change since that time has been an increased availability of information on nutrition and food content. As a result, people today can include a much wider variety of foods in the diet. This makes the diet more flexible and palatable than it was in Dr. Livingston's era. Following is an example of what two days' meal plans might look like for a child on the diet:

Breakfast
Scrambled egg with butter
Diluted cream
Orange juice

Breakfast
Bacon
Scrambled eggs with butter
Melon slices
Vanilla cream shake

Lunch
Spaghetti squash with butter
  and Parmesan cheese
Lettuce leaf with mayonnaise
Orange diet soda mixed with
  whipped cream

Lunch
Tuna with mayonnaise
Celery and cucumber sticks
Sugarless Jell-O with whipped cream

Dinner
Hot dog slices with catsup
Asparagus with butter
Chopped lettuce with mayonnaise
Vanilla cream popsicle

Dinner
Broiled chicken breast
Chopped lettuce with mayonnaise
Cinnamon apple slice with butter
  topped with vanilla ice cream

By identifying the four main food groups of the diet—protein, fruit or vegetable, fat, and cream—in each of these menus, you can begin to understand how the diet is constructed. This will be explained in greater detail later in the book.

The ketogenic diet must be calculated with precision, prepared meticulously using a gram scale, and followed rigidly.

To optimize the chance of success, the diet must be under-taken with the supervision of a dietitian trained in its use and a physician familiar with its many quirks. Even seemingly small mistakes, such as calculating too many calories into the diet, drinking too much water, or using medications that contain carbohydrates (even sunscreen!) can throw off the diet and perhaps bring on seizures.

Success on the ketogenic diet requires the commitment, determination, and faith of the entire family.

A ONE-MONTH TRIAL

Although the ketogenic diet must be calculated precisely and carefully weighed to the single gram, estimating the caloric needs of an individual, the basis for these rigorous calculations, remains an art form. Often a period of fine-tuning is needed before a child starts to reap the maximum benefits of the diet. For example, two children who are the same age, height, and weight may need very different numbers of calories on the diet (an active four-year-old requires more calories than one who is profoundly handicapped and does not even sit up). The dietitian cannot precisely assess a child's metabolic condition until after the diet is under way.

Some children need stricter limits on carbohydrate levels than others. Some have a difficult time with certain menus, or resist eating all the food at each meal. All of these points are worked out during the fine-tuning period.

For this reason, we ask parents, before starting the diet, to make a commitment to try their hardest for at least one month, preferably for three months.

The diet starts with the dietitian's and physician's best guess as to the correct diet prescription for a given child. But over the first month, or even the first three months, modifications will often be needed to help reach a diet plan that provides as much seizure control and satisfaction as possible for that individual child and family. The initiation of the diet in the hospital is too expensive and too time-consuming to waste on families who have not made a serious commitment. Initiating the diet requires a major commitment of time and energy on the part of the medical staff, which must be matched by an equal effort on the part of the child and family.

Virtually all children can stick to the diet—*IF* it is beneficial. Even before the diet begins, parents are encouraged to make sure that the child is enthusiastic about trying to get rid of his seizures and about trying to decrease the medicines. Parents can help a child to see how "tough" he is by asking him to give up his desserts and favorite snacks for two weeks. No desserts or snacks. This test is not the ketogenic diet, but it begins to prepare the child psychologically by approximating some of the sacrifices he will have to make in order to succeed on the diet. If the child does not want to do the diet, you cannot make him.

The one-month trial serves several purposes:

- In a single month doctors can usually ascertain if the diet is likely to be effective for a child. If the diet does not show *some* benefit in the first month, it is unlikely to work in the long run. If it does show benefit, fine-tuning over the next three months—and even six months—can often lead to even better seizure control and less medication.

- If the diet is working or shows potential to be effective within the first month, most families find that it is well worth the time and trouble to stick with it. Unlike the "honeymoon" effect of anticonvulsants, when many drugs work for just two weeks, it is relatively uncommon for the diet to work well for a period of time and then cease to work. Relapses are usually related to some change in circumstances, and control can usually be reestablished once the cause of the relapse has been identified.

- If the diet is not working after a month, or if it is not working sufficiently well after fine-tuning for three months, the family can always go back to trying to control the seizures through medication.

WHO IS A GOOD CANDIDATE FOR THE DIET?

Truthfully, it is not yet clear at what point in a person's epilepsy therapy the ketogenic diet should be considered. The family's psychology may be as relevant as the child's medical condition. In general, the diet has been reserved for children who have failed all anticonvulsant medications. This was an easy decision in the 1920s and 1930s when the only medications available were bromides and phenobarbital. As more anticonvulsant medicines became available, the ketogenic diet continued to be used as a last resort, reserved for when seizures remain incapacitating despite the use of two or three or more medications in combination.

Today there are so many anticonvulsant medications that they could be used in varying combinations and in increasing doses over years before all had been adequately tried. At Johns Hopkins our general guideline has been that a child continue to have at least two seizures per week despite the appropriate use of a minimum of two medications. This is an arbitrary definition, however, and the children we actually treat averaged more than 400 seizures per month despite having been on an average of more than six drugs. Despite this, more than half the children showed a dramatic decrease in their seizures.

Since the diet is so dramatically effective in this extreme population, perhaps it should be used earlier in the course of a child's difficult-to-control epilepsy, rather than merely as a last resort. Perhaps children should be considered as candidates for the diet as soon as a second medication fails to control their seizures. We have occasionally treated children whose seizures were controlled, but only with unacceptable side effects, with the aim of reducing or eliminating medications.

WHEN YOUR CHILD IS A ZOMBIE, when he sleeps practically the whole day and his eyes are glazed over, the whole family kind of feels sick. If you can get improvement with the diet, and the child starts being brighter and more responsive, the whole family feels better and breathes a sigh of relief. Even though weighing all the child's food and being tied down to strict meal plans is far from easy, it's worth it if you can improve the quality of life of your whole family. —LF

SEIZURE TYPES

The ketogenic diet may be tried on children with any type of seizure. Unlike anticonvulsant medication, it does not appear to have any adverse cognitive side effects. Even children with structural brain disorders such as microcephaly, hypoxic brain damage, prior strokes, and developmental abnormalities have had success with the diet. If a child has noticeably fewer seizures when sick or unable to eat, this may indicate potential for that child's success on the diet.

The outcomes for 150 children who were started on the diet at Johns Hopkins in 1996–1998 are shown in Table 1-1. Six months after starting the diet, 106 of the 150 children remained on it. Seizure type was not a strong predictor of seizure control on the diet.

The ketogenic diet appears particularly effective in controlling the myoclonic, absence, and atonic (drop) seizures associated with the Lennox-Gastaut syndrome. These are seizures that are particularly difficult to control with many of the older standard medications. The diet has also proven effective in children with both generalized tonic-clonic (grand mal) seizures and multifocal seizures. Our studies have shown that it is roughly equally effective in decreasing all types of seizures, but it remains our impression that the disabling "drop" seizures and myoclonic seizures, which often are most refractory to current anticonvulsant medications, appear to respond particularly well. Perhaps the diet's benefit in these seizures is most apparent because they occur so many times each day.

STRUCTURAL DISORDERS

Children whose seizures are due to structural lesions in the brain may also be candidates for the diet. Those whose seizures are the result of prenatal damage, birth asphyxia, or head trauma may all respond to the diet. We believe, but have not documented, that such children are somewhat less likely to achieve complete seizure control. We have had complete control in children who have had seizures due to cysts,

TABLE 1-1

Seizure Control After Six Months on Ketogenic Diet by Seizure Type

Seizure Type	Total	Infantile Spasms	Myoclonic	Atonic/Drops	Atypical/Absence	Tonic-Clonic	Tonic
Total N	106	13	28	17	15	11	6
# seizure-free	5 (3%)	1 (8%)*	1 (4%)	2 (12%)	0	1 (9%)	0
> 90% control	43 (29%)	4 (31%)	12 (43%)	8 (47%)	9 (60%)	3 (27%)	1 (17%)
50–90% control	29 (19%)	3 (23%)	8 (29%)	5 (30%)	2 (13%)	5 (45%)	2 (33%)
< 50% control	29 (19%)	5 (39%)	7 (25%)	2 (12%)	4 (27%)	2 (18%)	3 (50%)

Adapted from Freeman, Vining et al., *Pediatrics*, December 1998

Note: Percentages are of the most disabling seizure type in each child. A total of 106 patients were on the diet, but five patients' seizures were unclassifiable.

*Includes complex partial, simple partial, and partial with secondary generalization.

Sturge-Weber syndrome, and tuberous sclerosis, as well as in children with other focal cortical abnormalities.

When children with structural causes for their seizures are refractory to several medications, it may be reasonable to try the diet. However, if the diet is not successful within several months, and if the neurologic problem is amenable to surgery, then surgery may be the preferable alternative.

AGE

The ketogenic diet has been most often prescribed for children over one year of age. Children under the age of one year have been thought to have trouble becoming ketotic and maintaining ketosis. It has also been misbelieved that they would be prone to hypoglycemia. It turns out that neither of these beliefs is true. The diet has been successfully used in children as young as several months of age. It is important to remember that the diet requires careful and frequent supervision in young children who are actively growing and frequent modification as the child grows.

Traditionally the diet was rarely used in school-aged children because it was believed that their dietary habits were already too ingrained and that food temptations for children outside the home would be too great. An older child who already goes to school and loves McDonald's may find the diet more difficult than a very young child who has not yet formed strong eating habits. A child whose friends are eating pizza and cookies in the school cafeteria will be more tempted to cheat than one who spends all day with a parent. But in their determination to defeat their seizure disorders, older children can often summon up the willpower to resist temptation.

If they can bring their seizures under control, many children won't give up their ketogenic meals for anything. The strength and determination of many of these children amazes their parents and teachers.

Our studies of the effectiveness and the tolerability of the ketogenic diet in 150 consecutive children after one year, broken out by age group, is shown in Table 1-2. These studies reveal that the diet appears to work

TABLE 1-2

The Effect of Age on Outcomes of the Ketogenic Diet

Age at Start of Diet	# Initiating Diet	> 50% Improved Control at 12 Months
< 2 yrs	N = 27	59% (1 seizure-free)
2–5 yrs	N = 50	56% (4 seizure-free)
5–8 yrs	N = 32	50% (4 seizure-free)
8–12 yrs	N = 25	40% (1 seizure-free)
> 12 yrs	N = 16	31% (1 seizure-free)
Total	N = 150	50% (11 seizure-free)

Adapted from Freeman et al., *Pediatrics*, December 1998

equally effectively across different ages, and it is tolerated at each age—if it is effective.

KAY WAS A NORMAL FIVE-YEAR-OLD whose seizures had been uncontrollable before starting the diet several months earlier. One evening Kay's parents, who each worked two jobs, brought a pizza home for themselves and Kay's sister. Her father, intending to offer a piece to the sister, accidentally offered a piece to Kay instead. Her response was, "I can't have that, Daddy. I'm on a magic diet."

NOBODY THOUGHT THIS TEENAGER was going to stay on this diet. I am really amazed he has stuck to it as well as he has. He really fooled me. He used to snack constantly in front of the television. But by the time Brian started the diet, he was ready for it. He was 14 years old, really embarrassed by his seizures, and ready to try anything. Now he has no seizures and he wants to start going to school dances. I'm so proud of him. I can't believe it. —FD

The ketogenic diet works well in older children, provided that they and their families are highly motivated. Determined adolescents have completed the diet successfully. At the end of the day, motivation seems more important than age in determining the potential success of the diet.

ADULTS

Few adults have been tried on the diet, and it has never been offered to adults in a widespread, systematic fashion, nor have adults' responses to the diet been studied. Whether they can achieve as good ketosis and whether their seizures will be as well controlled remain to be researched. We know of no reason not to try the diet in adults *if* an experienced dietitian can be found who is willing to work with the adult and the physician.

> *AT FIRST WE DIDN'T GO OUT, even to my parents'. I was afraid of temptation, of making my son sad for what he couldn't have. But he missed the socializing. He said, "How come we never go out anymore?" I told him, "You couldn't order anything on the menu anyway." He said, "I could get ice for my ginger ale!" Now we go to a restaurant and take his meal with us. He tells the waitress, "I'm on a special diet so just bring me ice, please." —CC*

Megan and her parents met us for breakfast at the hotel when we were at a meeting in a nearby city. While we ordered breakfast, Megan asked the waitress for a cup of hot water for her tea and proceeded to unpack the ketogenic breakfast she had brought with her.

Most families find ways to integrate the diet into a happy, active life. Ingenuity, flexibility, good humor, and lack of self-pity go a long way toward making the diet acceptable to both the child and the family.

INTELLIGENCE

The level of a child's intelligence is not a criterion for selecting appropriate candidates for the diet. Some of the most dramatic successes have occurred in the most profoundly handicapped children. Other successes have occurred in children with normal intelligence. However, it is important for parents to carefully assess their goals and expectations before starting the diet. Parents may believe that their child's substantial intellectual delay is due solely to the medications, and that if they could only get their child off medication everything would be back to normal. Such parents are likely to be disappointed.

On the other hand, "electrical" seizures may be even more frequent than "clinical" seizures and may indeed interfere with intellect. Children with frequent myoclonic or "drop" seizures may have very chaotic EEGs and may have had intellectual deterioration since the start of their seizures. Such children may experience striking intellectual improvement if the diet is effective in controlling their seizures.

In short, the diet is intended primarily to control seizures. Decreasing and discontinuing medications is only a secondary goal. Improving intellect is a hope and a desire, but that is not what the ketogenic diet is designed to do.

NEW APPROACHES

This book is intended to help make the ketogenic diet available to the many families whose children are severely and profoundly handicapped by seizures or by the adverse side effects of current medications. Sometimes the ketogenic diet will free these children from both seizures and medications. When the diet is most effective, the children may after a time be "cured," in the sense that the diet may be slowly withdrawn and the children return to a normal diet while remaining seizure-free without medication.

When the first edition of this book was written in 1994, the ketogenic diet was considered by most members of the medical community to be an obscure and outdated mode of treatment. The first edition expressed the hope that future researchers, dietitians, epileptologists, neuroscientists, and parents would see for themselves that this diet can sometimes seem almost miraculous, allowing children plagued by a myriad of seizures to become seizure-free, and allowing children incapacitated by medications the freedom to develop to their full potential. We believed that seeing this with their own eyes, perhaps members of the medical community would begin to use modern technology to explore, and eventually to understand, the mechanisms involved. We hoped this would lead to the discovery of new approaches to seizure control—and seizure cure.

To a large extent our hopes and beliefs have begun to come true. Many medical centers are now offering the ketogenic diet. Some have begun systematically to study the diet's effectiveness and side effects. Some are asking questions about supplements with minerals and carnitine. The National Institutes of Health is supporting a double-blind study of the efficacy of the diet. Research is being conducted into the safety of the diet, into its effects on blood lipids, and the kidney stones that are its most common negative side effect. Laboratories are beginning to look at the metabolic and neurochemical effects of the diet in mice and rats in efforts to begin to learn how it might work. There is hope that future investigations of the diet may even lead to new approaches to conditions other than epilepsy.

The ketogenic diet has come a long way since *The Epilepsy Diet Treatment* was first published. Yet the journey to find a new, better, and easier approach to the treatment of difficult-to-control seizures has only just begun. As with most things in medicine, it is likely to be a long and arduous journey.

> **WHEN A PARENT CALLS UP** *and tells me a child hasn't had seizures in six months, that's the most wonderful news in the world.* —MK

HOW THE DIET WORKS

When parents come into the hospital with their children to initiate the diet, they learn that the body burns three types of fuel to produce energy. These fuel types are:

- CARBOHYDRATES: Starches, sugars, breads, cereal grains, fruits, vegetables

- FATS: Butter, margarine, oil, mayonnaise

- PROTEINS: Meat, fish, poultry, cheese, eggs, milk

Carbohydrates comprise approximately 50 percent to 60 percent of the average American's daily caloric intake. They are the least expensive and most efficient source of food energy. When carbohydrates are digested, the body converts them to glucose.

Glucose is the fuel source burned by the body to produce energy under normal circumstances. When its supply of glucose is limited, the body first burns adipose (fatty) tissue for energy. If caloric needs are not met by body fat, the body then draws from its protein stores (muscle), compromising good health. The body cannot store large amounts of glucose; it maintains only about a 24-hour supply. Fasting for 24 hours depletes body glucose. Once glucose is depleted, the body automatically draws on its other energy source—stored body fat.

In the absence of glucose, fat is not burned completely, but leaves a residue of "soot" or "ash" in the form of ketone bodies (acetone and acetoacetic acid). These ketone bodies build up in the blood. The ketogenic diet deliberately maintains this buildup of ketone bodies in the blood by forcing the body to burn fat, instead of glucose, as its primary source of energy. The ketones that are left from the burning of fat are *beta-hydroxybutyric acid* and *acetoacetate*. Beta-hydroxybutyric acid can be used by the liver and by the brain as a source of energy. Acetoacetic acid is excreted in the urine and imparts a sweet smell to the breath that has been likened to pineapple.

When ketone body levels are large enough, as indicated by a simple urine test, it is said that the body is "ketotic" (pronounced key-tah´-tic) or in a state of "ketosis." Ketosis is also evidenced, as mentioned above, by a fruity, sweet odor to the breath.

Fat energy is the basis of the ketogenic diet. In the presence of large levels of ketone bodies, seizures are frequently controlled. Unfortunately, we do not yet know precisely why the diet works. We will tell you what we do know in Chapter 3.

CHAPTER TWO

ANSWERS TO COMMON QUESTIONS

Q   *My child loves pizza and ice cream. Eating is an important part of our family life. How could we ever go on the diet successfully?*

A   If you are creative, you can find a way to adapt and still follow the diet. Pizza? Try a grilled tomato or eggplant slice topped with cheese—this becomes a ketogenic pizza. Ice cream? No problem! The cream in the diet can be frozen into scoops or popsicles, flavored with allowed sweeteners and baking chocolate, vanilla, or strawberries. The kind of pizza or ice cream your child is accustomed to having may seem unimportant when a "magic diet" helps to get rid of seizures!

Your child can go on the diet successfully because both of you want to cure the seizures. Much, perhaps most, of the diet's success will depend on your positive attitude and persuasiveness as a parent. If a parent does not have a positive attitude, the child will not cooperate and the diet will not work.

Q *Won't my child gain weight on all that fatty food?*

A On this diet the amount of food is carefully calculated so that your child will eat all the calories and protein needed for good health, but not so many that weight is gained. The fat content of the food has no bearing on weight as long as overall calories are strictly limited. Although restricting calories is important for achieving seizure control, calories will be adjusted up or down if weight gain or loss is recommended by the dietitian and physician, or if abnormal weight gain or loss occurs. It is normal for weight gain to accompany growth in height, but even this growth may be slowed while your child is on the diet. Height and weight will catch up when your child returns to a normal diet.

Q *Suppose my daughter eats a piece of toast. Will she go out of ketosis? Will I have to start over?*

A Yes, she may go out of ketosis, but you will not have to start over. You may, however, need to bring your child back into ketosis by skipping a meal or two until ketones in the urine reach the four-plus level, then start meals again as usual. If a mistake like this causes a breakthrough seizure, it will not spoil the long-term effects of the diet. Even so, loss of ketosis should be kept to a minimum.

Q *My child was seizure-free on the diet for three weeks but had a seizure yesterday. Why?*

A There are several potential causes of a breakthrough seizure in a child who has been well controlled on the diet. One cause is eating food that is not part of the meal plans. Family members and others often do not understand the need for strict compliance, and slip food to the child thinking they are being nice. Older and more mobile children are more likely to break the diet.

   Infections, kidney stones, and severe constipation are among other potential causes of breakthrough seizures. Incorrect preparation methods, such as purchasing a new commercial food product not calculated into a meal plan, can also lead to problems, as can medications containing glucose or carbohydrates. Illness might also cause breakthrough seizures in some children. If a breakthrough seizure occurs in a child who has been well controlled on the diet, it is almost always due to an aberration or mistake, and seizure control can easily be reestablished.

Q   *If my child has a seizure after being well controlled for three weeks on the diet, what should I do?*

A   Stay calm. Remember how far your child has come since starting on the diet. Then investigate to see if you can trace—and eliminate—the cause. First, check to see if your child ate something extra. Could a friend have offered a spare cookie? Might Grandma have slipped in a chocolate? Is the dog's food sealed tightly? Is the toothpaste missing? Have any new or different medicines or vitamin supplements been taken? Just a spoonful of regular cough syrup or "sugarless" foods containing sugar substitutes with carbohydrate, such as mannitol, sorbitol, polydextrose, or maltodextrin, can cause breakthrough seizures. We have even seen the sorbitol in suntan lotion cause breakthrough seizures.

Next, review your preparation methods. Did you do anything different? Did you weigh vegetables raw that should have been cooked? Buy a new brand of sausage? Measuring oil by volume instead of by weight could be a problem if you are using a large amount of oil. All food should be measured on a gram scale.

Is your child gaining weight? Weight gain is one sign that the diet is not being properly calculated or prepared. Seizures may continue or recur if the diet is providing more calories than your child's body needs to maintain itself. In such a case, the calorie count may need to be reduced slightly. Since every child's situation is different, you will need to do some sleuthing to solve the problem. Your doctor or dietitian may also be able to isolate the possible cause of seizures by listening to you and carefully reviewing your child's diet.

If your child was previously having frequent seizures and then was seizure-free for several weeks on the diet, the diet is likely to be effective despite the breakthrough seizures—it just needs fine-tuning.

Q   *I am doing everything my doctor told me but my child's seizures are continuing. What more can I do?*

A   Go over the diet and your home circumstances with a fine-tooth comb with your dietitian to be sure there are no mistakes in preparation or anyone giving unplanned food. Perhaps better seizure control could be achieved with fewer calories. Changing to a more restrictive 4.5:1 ratio of fat to protein plus carbohydrate for a few months may help. In some cases, a 5:1 ketogenic ratio is needed. Some children on the ketogenic diet will continue to have some seizures. The goal of the diet is to reduce the number and intensity of seizures as much as you can; complete control is not always possible. In the end it is up to you to decide whether the diet's rigor is worth the level of seizure control and freedom from medications that it provides your child. Some children's seizures do not respond or do not respond sufficiently well to continue the diet.

Q   *Is the ketogenic diet nutritionally complete?*
A   The ketogenic diet is nutritionally complete only when proper supplements are taken. Multivitamins, trace minerals, and calcium must be given as dietary supplements in sugar-free form. Some people ask whether carnitine should be added to the diet. We have conducted the diet for decades without carnitine, and no data indicate that it is necessary or useful as a supplement for all children. Because carnitine is expensive, we do not use it unless a child is weak and lacks energy *and* improves after taking carnitine. Some nutritionists have also claimed that the diet is deficient in trace minerals such as zinc and selenium. All we can say is that we have treated scores of children without any evidence of adverse effects

from the absence of micronutrients, but that the diet is indeed deficient in vitamins and minerals and must be supplemented.

Q   *What can my child eat at school?*

A   Your dietitian will help you plan meals that can easily be transported to school. Tuna, egg, or chicken salads are particularly easy to carry in Tupperware containers. Warm or chilled food can be carried in a small cooler or insulated bag, or wrapped in foil. Your child will have to learn to tell the teacher and classmates "No, thanks!" when snacks are distributed to the class. For occasions such as birthday parties, you can send your child to school with a container of special cheesecake or frozen eggnog (see Chapter 4) that can be eaten when the other kids eat their cake. It is remarkable how even young children of four or five years can learn to refuse treats, saying, "I'm a special kid on a special diet."

Q   *Can we go to a restaurant or on a day's outing while my child is on the diet?*

A   With imagination, planning, and persistence, you and your child can go anywhere on the diet. On short trips, you can take one or more pre-prepared meals in a cooler. You can ask to have a pre-prepared meal heated in a restaurant's microwave. Ketogenic eggnog or macadamia nuts (sometimes mixed with calculated butter) can serve as occasional easy meal replacements, for instance if you are in transit at mealtime.

Q   *Can we still go on family trips?*

A   You may go on longer trips if all the ingredients of your child's diet are under your control. You can stay in a hotel or motel with a kitchenette, where you can prepare your own or your child's meals. You can order plain grilled chicken, steamed vegetables or fresh fruit, butter, and heavy whipping cream at a restaurant, and weigh portions on your scale when the food arrives. Remember, though, that tiny bits of extra foods such as catsup, dill pickle, or lemon juice can upset your child's ketosis if they are not calculated into the meal. For greater detail on how to preserve your mobility while on the diet, see Chapter 6.

Q *The amounts of food allowed in the diet are so small—won't my child feel hungry?*

A Ketosis suppresses appetite, so children on the diet are not usually as hungry as other children. The diet is hypocaloric, providing only about three-quarters of the calories that would normally be recommended for a child's height and weight. However, ketosis and the concentration of fat in the diet help to create a full feeling in the stomach despite the small quantity of food. Some children feel hungry for the first week or two of the diet, but their stomachs usually adjust with time. More food may decrease ketosis and actually increase the child's hunger.

Q *What if my child refuses to eat all the food in a meal?*

A Because of the small quantity, children usually need to eat all of the food on the diet in order to feel full. If your child does refuse food, however, you must use your powers of persuasion and try to create a menu that might be more acceptable for the next meal. The key to success is to be creative, not rigid, within the bounds of the diet. Ultimately, to provide proper nutrition and maintain ketosis, all of the food in a meal must be consumed at one time—it may not be saved until the next meal or eaten between meals. If ketosis is not maintained, the diet will not work.

EATING IT ALL

There are few things in a child's life that she can control. Eating is one of them. You, the parent, are in a difficult position with the ketogenic diet. You are told that the child must eat everything on her plate. What if she refuses? Give her approximately 20 minutes to eat her meal. If she hasn't eaten, then throw it away and wait for the next meal. If you are placed in the position of coaxing or wheedling your child into eating "just two more bites," you will lose. On occasion we have seen parents placed in the position where every meal is a battle that extends from one meal to the next. We have even seen a mother finally hire a sitter just to feed the child (in 20 minutes) and break the pattern. The diet goes more smoothly when parents learn to be more relaxed about feeding and children learn that they are not ultimately in control.

Q   *My daughter is doing so well on the diet. She has had no seizures. But there is a flu going around and she vomited all last evening. This afternoon her ketones are low. Why? What should I do?*

A   The low ketones may well be due to the infection and the alterations in her metabolism caused by her illness. Since she has been doing so well on the diet, you should probably do nothing. She will most likely be back to eating by morning. In the meantime, you should make sure she gets enough liquid to stay hydrated. If she has stopped vomiting, you might try offering sips of her ketogenic eggnog; since every sip is balanced in terms of its ketogenic ratio, it does not matter if your child only drinks a little bit.

   If dehydration becomes a problem, it may be necessary to give some Pedialyte (a chemically balanced fluid available at the drugstore). Pedialyte contains about 23 grams of carbohydrate per 1,000 cc. When the child is not eating any food, the carbohydrate in Pedialyte often is no greater than the combined protein and carbohydrate allotment in the diet, so Pedialyte often does not upset ketosis. In case of severe dehydration, it may be necessary to get an intravenous saline solution at the hospital. Intravenous dextrose should not be used because it will upset ketosis.

Q   *What if my daughter has a seizure while she is sick with the flu?*

A   Illness may sometimes cause a transient drop in ketone levels. If your daughter starts to have seizures during an illness, following recovery you can put her on a fast for one to three meals until she goes back into ketosis, and then restart the diet, perhaps at half quantity for a few meals. The effectiveness of the diet is only partly represented by high levels of ketones in the urine. Some children have seizures even while their urinary ketones remain high, while others may do well despite a transient drop in ketones. The most important measure is how well the child is doing.

Q *My son got bronchitis and his doctor prescribed an antibiotic. How do I know if this will affect the diet?*

A All medicines and pharmaceuticals, from toothpaste to cough syrup to vitamins to prescription medicine, must, *whenever possible,* be free of all sugar and carbohydrate. Some common forms of sugar and carbohydrate to watch out for on labels are glucose, sucrose, fructose, dextrose, sorbitol, and mannitol. Medication in chewable or tablet form often contains some carbohydrate to bind the tablet together, and sweet-tasting elixirs or syrups often contain sugar. Ask your doctor to prescribe needed medications in sugar-free and carbohydrate-free forms. If you have questions, the best source of information is your pharmacist. In fact, a pharmacist is often an important part of the ketogenic diet team, helping parents through their child's illnesses throughout the duration of the diet. If your pharmacist cannot help, go directly to the manufacturer. Formulas often change; read labels carefully and don't take anything for granted.

In an emergency, or if it is not possible to find a sugar-free formula, take care of your child's health first. If losing ketosis is a price that must be paid for your child's health, then after the illness your child can always fast again and reinstitute the diet. (See Appendix A on medications for more detail.)

Q *The ketogenic diet is making my child constipated. How do I keep this from being a problem?*

A Constipation is the most common problem we see in children on the diet. Here are a few anticonstipation measures you can try:

- Use meal plans that contain as much fiber as possible. You are allowed to use two lettuce leaves, or about one-half cup of chopped lettuce, per day as a "free" food, and you can use calculated mayonnaise as dressing. Using more Group A vegetables can also help, since you can serve twice as many of these as of Group B vegetables.

- Try cutting out meal plans with catsup, chocolate, or other carbohydrate-based flavorings that take away from the quantity of fiber-rich vegetables your child can eat.

- In extreme cases, you can use a stool softener such as Colace or a gentle laxative such as Milk of Magnesia, diluted Baby Fleet enemas, or other children's rectal suppositories. One mother used a diluted enema regularly every other day, pouring out two-thirds of the dosage so the long-term use would not hurt her son's bowels. MCT oil, in small amounts, may be calculated into the diet to relieve constipation. (For more on constipation see Chapter 5.)

Q *Is it possible for my child to become too ketotic?*

A Yes. The level of ketone bodies may become unusually high and your child may experience shallow, panting breathing, but this is rare. If this happens, give him a sip of orange juice or a cracker to bring the ketone levels back in the normal high ketone range. If your child becomes both too ketotic and too dehydrated (not taking enough fluid and not passing enough urine), the physician or the hospital may have to give some fluids intravenously. They may, if necessary, give a small amount of glucose. When your child perks up, the diet can be resumed. If excess ketosis becomes a recurring problem, the dietitian can try reducing the child's ketogenic ratio to 3:1.

CHAPTER THREE

AN HISTORICAL OVERVIEW OF THE KETOGENIC DIET

Thirty grams cream, 12 grams meat, 18 grams butter—the recipe begins to sound like old witches concocting a magic brew. There is mystery to it. No one understands exactly how or why the ketogenic diet works. But it *does* work, and it has worked for more than 75 years.

Studies conducted from the 1920s to the 1980s showed that:

- The diet completely controlled epilepsy in one-third of the children whose seizures were otherwise uncontrollable.

- In half of the remaining children, the diet markedly decreased the frequency of seizures and/or enabled medications to be reduced.

- Many children whose seizures had been completely controlled could return to a normal diet in two to three years and remain seizure-free without medication. They had either been cured of epilepsy or had recovered from their previously uncontrollable epilepsy.

- Permanent seizure control often began within days of diet initiation.

These results come from different eras; from times when there were far fewer anticonvulsants available and from times when studies were conducted with less rigor and were often based on retrospective data analysis. More recent studies of the diet's efficacy and tolerability show that almost one-third of children starting on the diet have their seizures virtually (more than 90 percent) controlled. Despite the dramatic advances in our understanding of epilepsy and neurophysiology, and despite the large number of new anticonvulsant medications now available, the diet remains surprisingly effective in a large percentage of children with difficult-to-control seizures.

HISTORY OF THE KETOGENIC DIET[1]

Fasting has been used as a treatment for seizures and epilepsy since biblical times and is mentioned again in the literature of the Middle Ages. However, it wasn't until the 1921 American Medical Association convention, at which Rawle Geylin, a prominent New York pediatrician, reported the successful treatment of severe epilepsy by fasting, that interest began to reawaken. Geylin cited the case of a "child of a friend. . . ," age 10, who ". . . for four years had had grand mal and petit mal attacks which had become practically continuous." At Battle Creek he came under the care of an osteopath, (Dr. Hugh Conklin), who promptly fasted him, the first fast being one of 15 days. There were several subsequent periods of feeding then fasting. "After the second day of fasting," Geylin reports, "the epileptic attacks ceased and he had no attacks in the ensuing year." Geylin reported seeing two other patients, also treated by Dr. Conklin, who after fasting had been seizure-free for two and three years. He further reported that he had fasted 26 of his own

---

[1]This section is adapted from *The Ketogenic Diet—1997* by Swink T, Vining EPG, and Freeman JM, *Advances in Pediatrics* 44; 297–329, *The Annual Review of Pediatrics,* Mosby-Yearbook, 1977. Complete references may be found there.

patients with epilepsy. Six patients showed no improvement and 18 showed marked improvement. Two remained seizure-free for more than one year. Dr. Geylin stated that the best length of fasting was 20 days. This was the first American report of the benefits of fasting on epilepsy.

Dr. Conklin, believing that epilepsy was caused by intoxication of the brain from substances coming from the Peyer's patches of the intestine, developed his "fasting treatment" program to put the patient's intestine at complete rest. He stated, "I deprive the patient of all food, giving nothing but water over as long a period of time as he is physically able to stand it. . . . Some will fast for twenty-five days and come to the office one or more times every day for (osteopathic) treatment. . . ."

Dr. William Lennox, considered by many to be the father of American pediatric epilepsy, relates Conklin's fasting treatment to the origin of the ketogenic diet. According to Lennox, who later reviewed Geylin's records, long-term freedom from seizures occurred in 15 of 79 of Geylin's fasted children (18 percent). The father of Hugh Conklin's patient reported by Geylin was Charles Howland, a wealthy New York corporate lawyer, and the boy's uncle was Dr. John Howland, Professor of Pediatrics at the Johns Hopkins Hospital and Director of the newly opened Harriet Lane Home for Invalid Children at Hopkins in Baltimore. In 1919, Charles Howland gave his brother $5,000 to find out if there was a scientific basis for the success of the starvation treatment in his son. These funds were used to create the first American laboratories to study fluid and electrolyte balances in fasting children.

During the early 1920s, when only phenobarbital and bromides were available as antiseizure medications, reports that fasting could cure seizures were exciting and promised hope for children with epilepsy. These reports set off a flurry of clinical and research activity.

This was also an era of early investigations and understanding of the metabolic basis for diabetes and for the often-fatal ketoacidosis that accompanied diabetes. A 1921 review article about diabetes and its dietary management stated that ". . . acetone, acetic acid, and ß-hydroxy-butyric acid appear (even) . . . in a normal subject (caused) by starvation, or a diet containing too low a proportion of carbohydrate and too high a proportion of fat. [ketoacidosis] appears to be the immediate result of the oxidation of certain fatty acids in the absence of a sufficient proportion of 'oxidizing' (dissociated) glucose."

DISCOVERY OF THE KETOGENIC DIET

The first article suggesting that a diet high in fat and low in carbohydrate might simulate the metabolic effects of starvation was published in 1921. Wilder, its author, proposed that, "the benefits of fasting could be . . . obtained if ketonemia was produced by other means. . . ." Ketone bodies are formed from fat and protein whenever a disproportion exists between the amount of fatty acid and the amount of sugar. "It is possible," Wilder wrote, "to provoke ketogenesis by feeding diets which are rich in fats and low in carbohydrates. It is proposed to try the effects of such diets on a series of epileptics. . . ." The calculation of such a diet, and the effectiveness of Wilder's proposed "ketogenic" diet, was reported in 1924 from the Mayo Clinic by Peterman. Peterman's diet used 1 gram of protein per kilogram of body weight in children (less in adults), 10–15 grams of carbohydrate per day, and the remainder of the calories as fat. The individual's caloric requirement was calculated based on the basal metabolic rate plus 50 percent.[2] It is virtually identical to the ketogenic diet that is used today. Of the first 17 patients treated by Peterman with this new

---

[2]The ketogenic diet as developed by Wilder and a fellow diabetologist at the Mayo Clinic is based on the concept that some foods are more likely to increase the body's production of ketone bodies, while others are "anti-ketogenic." Any glucose will exert an anti-ketogenic effect because it is completely burned by the body. A small portion of ingested fat (1 part of 10), a significant part of the protein (more than half), and all carbohydrates are broken down to glucose and are anti-ketogenic. This has been expressed in the formula:

$$\frac{\text{Ketogenic}}{\text{Anti-Ketogenic}} = \frac{K}{AK} = \frac{0.9 \text{ Fat} + 0.46 \text{ Protein}}{1.0 \text{ Carbohydrate} + 0.1 \text{ Fat} + 0.58 \text{ Protein}}$$

The ketogenic:anti-ketogenic ratio of food in a diet must be at least 1.5:1 to produce noticeably elevated levels of ketone bodies in the blood and urine. Seizure control is best when the ratio is at least 3:1. Calories must be limited to maintain ketosis.

diet, 10 (59 percent) became seizure-free, 9 on the diet alone. Four others (23 percent) had marked improvement, two were lost to follow-up, and one discontinued the diet. The following year he reported 37 patients treated over a period of 2.5 years: 19 (51 percent) were seizure-free, and 13 (35 percent) were markedly improved. These initial reports were rapidly followed by others from many centers. The currently used protocol for calculating and initiating the ketogenic diet is well discussed by Talbot in 1927.

Reports of the effectiveness of the diet appeared throughout the late 1920s and 1930s. In these reports, subjects varied and patients were followed up for varying lengths of time. As shown in Table 3-1, 60 percent to 75 percent of children generally had a greater than 50 percent decrease in their seizures, 30 percent to 40 percent of these had a greater than 90 percent decrease in the seizure frequency, and 20 percent to 30 percent had little or no seizure control.

The ketogenic diet was widely used throughout the 1930s because no new effective medications had been developed. When diphenyl-

TABLE 3-1

Seizure Control with the Ketogenic Diet:
Reports from the Literature 1925–1986*

Author	Year	No. of Patients	Seizure Control		
			> 90%	50–90%	< 50%
Peterman	1925	36	51%	35%	23%
Helmholtz	1927	91	31%	23%	46%
Wilkens	1937	30	24%	21%	50%
Livingston	1954	300	43%	34%	22%
Kinsman	1992	58	29%	38%	33%
Huttenlocher—MCT	1971	12	—	50%	50%
Trauner—MCT	1985	17	29%	29%	42%
Sills et al.—MCT	1986	50	24%	20%	56%

*Representative studies

Note: MCT = Medium-chain triglyceride diet

hydantoin was discovered in 1939, the attention of physicians and researchers turned from the mechanisms of action and efficacy of the diet to new anticonvulsants. A new era of medication treatment for epilepsy had begun. Compared with medication, the diet was thought to be relatively difficult, rigid, and expensive.

As new anticonvulsant medications became available, the diet was used less frequently. As fewer children were placed on the ketogenic diet, fewer dietitians were trained in the rigors and nuances of the "classic" ketogenic diet. Therefore, the diets were often less precise, less rigorous, and so less ketogenic and less effective than they had been in previous years. A form of the diet was developed using medium-chain triglyceride (MCT) oil. This oil was more ketogenic and allowed larger portions of food, but children on the MCT diet often suffered from nausea, diarrhea, and bloating; therefore, despite the decrease in seizures, parents often found the side effects unacceptable and gave up. Schwartz and colleagues in Oxford, England, conducted the only comparative trial of the various diets that had been developed. Testing the classic ketogenic diet, the MCT diet, and a "modified" MCT diet, their study (Table 3-2) showed that 41 percent of patients had a greater than 90 percent seizure reduction. No one diet was superior to others. The MCT diet was found unpalatable by more children, and diarrhea and vomiting were more common on the MCT diet. Experiences like these

TABLE 3-2

Comparison of Clinical Response to Various Ketogenic Diets

	Reduction in Seizure Frequency		
Diet (59 individuals)*	> 90%	50–90%	< 50%
Classic 4:1 (N = 24)	11	11	2
MCT (N = 27)	10	11	6
Radcliffe (N = 12)	5	3	4
N studies (N = 63)	26 (41%)	25 (40%)	12 (19%)

Adapted from Schwartz et al., *Dev Med Child Neurol* 1989; 31:145–151.

*Some who failed one diet were tried on another.

led to the widespread opinion that diet treatment for epilepsy did not work or was very difficult to tolerate.

Even today, although we understand considerably more about the neurochemistry and neurophysiology of epilepsy, we do not understand why most seizures start or why they stop. We do not understand what factors initiate a seizure, the mechanisms by which seizures are stopped, or what inhibits some from spreading. We know some of the neurochemistry and physiologic events that accompany the electrical discharges of single cells and are only beginning to study the interactions of cellular populations. We know some of the chemistry and physiologic effects of medications, but we still do not know how they work.

In 1992, Charlie Abrahams, age 2, developed multiple myoclonic seizures, generalized tonic and tonic-clonic seizures, refractory to many medications. "Thousands of seizures and countless medications later, after five pediatric neurologists, two homeopathic physicians, one faith healer, and one fruitless surgery, Charlie's seizures remained unchecked and his prognosis was for continued seizures and progressive retardation," wrote Jim Abrahams, Charlie's father.

Searching for answers on his own, Charlie's father found reference to the ketogenic diet and to Johns Hopkins. Charlie was brought to Johns Hopkins, where the diet had continued to be used, and he was started on the diet. His seizures were completely controlled, his EEG returned to normal, his development resumed, and he no longer suffered the side effects of medication. Charlie's father wanted to know why no one had told him about the diet before. He found references to the high success rates discussed previously and determined that this information should be readily available so that other parents could become aware of the ketogenic diet. Creating the Charlie Foundation, Charlie's father, a filmmaker and fund-raiser, used his talents to produce videos, fund the initial publication of this book, and underwrite conferences to train physicians and dietitians from medical centers nationwide. Many medical centers began to use the diet. (After Charlie remained seizure-free for two years, he was allowed to come off the diet. Several months later he had a few further seizures. Since resuming the diet in January 1996, he has remained medication-free and virtually seizure-free on a modified form of the ketogenic diet.)

With the help of the Charlie Foundation, the use and awareness of the ketogenic diet expanded dramatically. Charlie Abrahams's story was covered on national television and magazines, further raising awareness of the diet.

The history of this rapid expansion in use and awareness is well described by Wheless, who concluded in 1995 that the ketogenic diet compares favorably with other new treatments for epilepsy in children. The diet offers a far greater chance for seizure control than any of the anticonvulsant medicines developed in the past 50 years.

Prospective studies evaluating the effectiveness of the ketogenic diet are now becoming available. A 1998 multicenter study of 51 children who averaged 230 seizures per month before starting the diet (Table 3-3) documented that almost half (45 percent) remained on the diet for one year, and almost half of those (43 percent) remaining on the diet (Column B) were virtually seizure-free. Eighty-three percent of those remaining on the diet for one year had better than a 50 percent decrease in their seizures.

TABLE 3-3

Outcomes of the Ketogenic Diet: A Multicenter Study (N = 51)

	Number (%) of Those on Diet		By Intention to Treat	
Seizure Control	A 6 months	B 12 months	C 6 months	D 12 months
	N = 34 (66%) on diet	N = 23 (45%) on diet	N = 34 (66%) on diet	N = 23 (45%) on diet
> 90% (# seizure-free)	n = 14 (41%) (6)	n = 10 (43%) (5)	n = 14 (27%) (6)	n = 10 (20%) (5)
50–90%	n = 12 (35%)	n = 9 (39%)	n = 12 (24%)	n = 9 (18%)
< 50%	n = 8 (24%)	n = 4 (17%)	n = 8 (16%)	n = 4 (8%)
Discontinued diet	n = 16	n = 27	n = 16	n = 27
Patients missing	n = 1	n = 1	n = 1	n = 1

Vining et al., *Annals of Neurology*, December 10, 1998

This multicenter study also shows the difficulties of comparing new studies with older ones, which used a different approach to reporting their outcomes. If you look at this same multicenter study from a different angle and include all of those children that the centers "intended to treat," meaning everyone who was started on the diet even if they only remained on it for a day or a week, then, as is shown in columns C and D, the same 45 percent of the children remained on the diet for 12 months. But only 10 (20 percent) of those starting on the diet had better than 90 percent seizure control at one year, and an additional nine children (18 percent) had a 50 percent to 90 percent decrease in seizures.

This newer "intention to treat" way of reporting clinical trials of treatment gives a better concept of the chance of a treatment being effective. If we "intend to treat" a child with the ketogenic diet, the chance of decreasing that child's seizures by more than 90 percent are one in four, according to this methodology.

Between 1994 and 1999 we have started more than 400 children on the diet at Johns Hopkins. The outcomes of 150 consecutive children are shown in Table 3-4. Before starting the diet, these children averaged more than 600 seizures per month and had been on an average of more than six medications.

 TABLE 3-4

Outcomes of the Ketogenic Diet: Johns Hopkins Patients, 1998

Number Initiating	Seizure Control and Diet Status	Time After Starting the Diet		
		3 months	6 months	12 months
Total N=150	100% seizure-free	4 (3%)	5 (3%)	11 (7%)
	> 90%	46 (31%)	43 (29%)	30 (20%)
	50–90%	39 (26%)	29 (19%)	34 (23%)
	< 50%	36 (24%)	29 (19%)	8 (5%)
	Continued on diet	125 (83%)	106 (71%)	83 (55%)
	Discontinued diet	25 (17%)	44 (29%)	67 (45%)

Freeman et al., *Pediatrics* 11/98

SUMMARY OF RESULTS

As Table 3-4 shows, even among children who cannot be helped by modern anticonvulsant medications:

- Twenty-seven percent have had their seizures virtually controlled.
- Half (50 percent) of the children treated with the ketogenic diet had better than a 50 percent decrease in their seizures.
- Seven percent of these children were free of seizures within one year after starting on the ketogenic diet.
- An additional 20 percent of those starting on the diet had a more than 90 percent reduction in seizures as measured at the end of one year.

It is notable that virtually all of those remaining on the diet for one year had at least a 50 percent decrease in seizures. Those who had less than a 50 percent reduction often decided that the diet was too much trouble and discontinued it. It is also noteworthy that most of the children who had success with the diet had shown some success during the first three months. The degree of success might improve after three months, but if there was not a 50 percent decrease in seizures during that time, it was less likely to occur in subsequent months.

THEORETICAL BASIS OF THE KETOGENIC DIET

How does the diet work? We wish that we knew. We know that the body is able to burn fats as a source of energy and that the brain is able to use the ketone bodies left over as its own energy source. It appears that a high level of ketones provides better seizure control, and we know that even small amounts of carbohydrate can quickly break the ketosis and may result in seizures. We also know that in some children the seizures can be completely controlled and those children may after a time slowly discontinue the diet, often with no return of the seizures.

However, while it appears that ketones suppress seizures and carbohydrate interferes with this suppression, at present we do not know the mechanisms involved. Understanding how the diet works will also require more information about seizures and epilepsy, and at present we know remarkably little about either.

While the short answer to the question "How does the ketogenic diet work?" is "We don't really know," the longer answer is that there may be a combination of factors at work:

KETONE BODIES come in many chemical forms and are the result of the incomplete burning of fats in the body. They have both a sedative effect and an appetite-suppressing effect. Some popular weight-reduction diets with very low calorie levels and low carbohydrates produce ketosis and use the appetite-suppressing effect of ketosis to prevent the dieter from feeling too hungry.

Ketone bodies also have an anticonvulsant effect. For example, seizures may occur when a child whose seizures are well controlled on the diet eats a cookie—even if urinary ketones are not clearly affected. While the concentration of ketones in the blood is more important than that in the urine, ketones are measured in the urine for convenience. If there are no ketones in the urine, the diet is not going to work. But even if the ketones in the urine are strong, sometimes the diet can be made more effective with a higher ratio of fats to protein and carbohydrates, or with fewer calories.

Three to four plus ketones in the urine are necessary—although not sufficient—for good seizure control. The ketones most relevant to seizure control are probably those in the brain, but sampling brain ketone levels is not currently possible. The ketones in the blood are a much closer approximation of the ketones in the brain than are those in the urine. Sampling of blood has in the past been expensive and has required a needle stick. We are currently studying the ability to measure blood ketones by finger stick, as is done routinely today by diabetic patients measuring their own blood sugar levels. When a reliable method of easily and cheaply measuring serum ketones at home exists, the goal of fine-tuning the diet probably will focus more on producing the optimal levels of serum ketones. At this point it can only be speculated that an ability to track daily ketone levels in the blood will further improve our ability to control seizures.

ACIDOSIS means an increased amount of acid in the blood. Ketone bodies are acids and therefore cause acidosis. There are several other chemical mechanisms by which the human body produces acidosis and many ways in which the body compensates for the ketones to maintain a normal pH (acid/base) balance. Acidosis influences the threshold for seizures. This is why seizures can be reduced temporarily by the ingestion of acids or acid-forming salts, or breathing a mixture high in carbon dioxide. Hyperventilating, which blows off the carbon dioxide, reduces acidosis and can bring out absence seizures. Acidosis may be one of the participants facilitating seizure control in the ketogenic diet, but since the body quickly compensates for the acidosis to readjust its pH balance, it cannot be the major determinant of the diet's success.

DEHYDRATION was part of the original water diet used by McFadden that ultimately led to the development of the ketogenic diet. While fluids are traditionally limited during the diet, the role, if any, of dehydration in seizure control is unclear. It is known that administering excess water can provoke seizures, probably due to acute dilution of the body's sodium level. Indeed, this was one of the methods used in the past by physicians to provoke seizures for observation. However, this in no way indicates that dehydration would prevent seizures by raising the body's sodium level. Normal kidneys do an excellent job of maintaining the body's chemical balance.

Another misconception about fluid intake is that fluid dilutes the ketones, thereby negating the effects of the ketogenic diet. Increased water intake certainly results in urine that is more dilute. If the body's production and excretion of ketones is constant, the concentration of ketones in the urine (and therefore the strength of the urinary ketone test) will depend on the child's water intake. This does not, however, necessarily reflect the level of ketones in the blood and brain, which may be higher. Water intake is limited on the ketogenic diet because this appears, in practice, to improve seizure control. The underlying reasons for this are still little understood. Too much fluid restriction may lead to kidney stone formation (discussed later).

None of the individual mechanisms discussed here will, in isolation, lead to seizure control, since the body can compensate for each of them. Acidosis corrects itself in one to two weeks, and the pH of the blood will remain normal throughout the remainder of the diet. Changes in the water and electrolyte content of the brain are rapidly compensated for by the rest of the body.

OTHER INFLUENCES ON METABOLISM are probably keys to the real effectiveness of the diet. For example, while the brains of children and adults burn glucose almost exclusively, the fetus and newborn are able to exist on a metabolism of fats. Does the ketogenic diet enable the brain to revert to a more primitive form of metabolism? Is the reason that the ketogenic diet may be more effective in children than in adults based on the younger brain's capability to metabolize fats? There is also some suggestion that a diet that results in incompletely burned fats—ketones—particularly beta-hydroxybutyrate, may alter the chemistry of brain cell membranes and thereby the sensitivity of certain transmitter sites. Clearly, more research is needed to explore the mechanisms by which the ketogenic diet achieves its dramatic results.

THE NEED FOR RESEARCH

In the early 1960s Dr. H. Houston Merritt, codiscoverer of Dilantin and then director of the Neurologic Institute at the Columbia Presbyterian Medical Center in New York, told his residents that the discovery of Dilantin was a major setback to the understanding of epilepsy. At the time the effectiveness of Dilantin was discovered in the late 1930s, many people were investigating brain metabolism in epilepsy and beginning to study the mechanisms by which the ketogenic diet stopped seizures.

Since the discovery of Dilantin, however, efforts have been directed toward finding other drugs that would be equally effective, and few have gone back to look at the basic mechanisms by which the diet alters the brain's metabolism.

However, during the past few years many new studies of the diet have been launched. Studies with mice are showing that ketogenic food can induce ketosis in the animals and can raise their threshold for seizures. Other studies are questioning the effect of caloric restriction on seizure control.

Another study using mice involves infusing beta-hydroxybutyric acid (BOHB) to decrease the animals' seizures. These are some of the first attempts to measure the effects of BOHB on the brain of laboratory animals. Perhaps they will lead to understanding of how the diet works and how it affects seizures and epilepsy.

With new imaging techniques we can conduct studies in the same child under conditions of starvation and during initiation of the ketogenic diet, during seizures and between seizures. We could analyze acute changes in metabolism and evaluate longer-term changes in brain energy metabolism with continuation of the diet. We could use children for whom the diet is unsuccessful as controls to compare with those in whom the diet stops seizures. We can even use the same child as his or her own control by giving a small dose of glucose to a child whose seizures are well controlled on the diet and then studying any alterations in brain metabolism that take place subsequently. Through studies such as these, and others, we can hope to improve understanding in the future of why and through what mechanisms the ketogenic diet works.

Whatever the mechanisms of action of the ketogenic diet, they are likely to be different from the mechanisms of action of the drugs we currently use. The diet's effectiveness in varying seizure types and its action across varied ages suggests that its basis of action will be different from that of most current anticonvulsant drugs. If and when we understand how the ketogenic diet works, then perhaps we will also understand more about epilepsy itself.

USE OF THE KETOGENIC DIET: A PHYSICIAN'S VIEW

As discussed previously, pediatric neurologists in most of the world are now aware of the ketogenic diet. Unfortunately, despite all of the newer medications, there remain a lot of children with difficult to control epilepsy. If a child has failed two medications used appropriately and in combination, there is only a 15 percent to 20 percent chance of controlling that child's seizures with the addition of *any* further medications. The new medications may decrease the frequency of seizures in adults when they are tested, but few give more than a 50 percent decrease in seizures and complete control is rare. The chance of dramatic success with the newer medications is even less in difficult-to-control populations. Any patient who uses more than two anticonvulsants simultaneously dramatically increases the chance of side effects. Therefore, adding a third or fourth medication is likely to result in a child or adult who is toxic from medications and who also has continuing seizures.

The diet *is* a lot of trouble. No one would dispute that. But if it works, if it decreases seizures by more than 50 percent, or if it allows a substantial decrease in medication toxicity, it not only becomes tolerable but also "amazing," "fantastic," "a miracle," as can be loudly heard from the parents of children for whom it has been successful. If it doesn't work, parents can always go back to trying more or newer medications.

THE MEDIUM-CHAIN TRIGLYCERIDE (MCT) DIET

"WE HAVE ALREADY BEEN ON THE KETOGENIC DIET ONCE. We used that MCT oil stuff, and it was awful. Our daughter had terrible diarrhea and the seizures didn't improve, so we stopped after two weeks. Why would you suggest that we consider trying it again?" —TP

In the belief that the ketogenic diet was an effective form of therapy and that more families would try—and benefit from—a ketogenic diet if it were formulated with foods more closely approximating a normal diet, Dr. Peter Huttenlocher of the University of Chicago and his colleagues devised a diet that they believed would be more palatable than the "classic" ketogenic diet. They hoped that it would therefore foster compliance, while maintaining ketosis. They called their formulation the MCT diet, replacing the long-chain fats of the classic ketogenic diet with medium-chain triglycerides, which have shorter molecular chain lengths than the long-chain triglycerides found in cream, butter, and most other dietary fats. MCT comes as an odorless, colorless, tasteless oil. It is to be calculated into the diet, not merely poured on food.

An MCT diet with calories at 100 percent of RDA levels, and with more carbohydrates and protein, will produce the same urinary ketosis as a classic ketogenic diet with calories at 75 percent of RDA levels. MCT oil can thus be said to be more ketogenic than other dietary fats. Because the diet is more ketogenic, a child on the MCT diet can eat a wider variety of anti-ketogenic foods, such as larger portions of fruit and vegetables and even a small amount of bread and other starches. Fluids are not restricted on this diet.

The MCT diet, like the classic ketogenic diet, is initiated after a brief fast and usually shows results within several days of its inception. Children must stick with it rigidly, as with the classic ketogenic diet. If the MCT diet works, children similarly stay on it for about two years.

A comparison of the classic ketogenic diet with the MCT diet and a modified ketogenic diet (Table 3-2) found all three to be equally effective in achieving seizure control. Compliance and palatability, however, were found to be better with the classic ketogenic diet.

Although the MCT diet has been reported to be equally as effective as the classic ketogenic diet, this has not been our experience at Johns Hopkins. We have found that the MCT diet is usually too high in calories (thus providing inferior seizure control) and is not more palatable than the classic diet. In fact, our experience indicates that ingestion of the MCT oil is often accompanied by abdominal cramps, severe and persistent diarrhea, or nausea and vomiting. If children cannot hold it down, it cannot be effective. We will often supplement the "classic" ketogenic diet with small amounts of MCT oil, both because it can increase ketosis and because it may decrease the constipation that often accompanies the ketogenic diet.

Some parents or physicians may want to try the MCT diet for children, perhaps with the thought of providing a higher volume of food. If the child does not have trouble with the oil and if the seizures are completely controlled, some families appreciate the additional anti-ketogenic calories that the MCT diet affords. If the MCT diet does not work or if it is not tolerated, we recommend trying the classic ketogenic diet.

Many parents tell us that their child has already been on the ketogenic diet without success. On further questioning, this prior diet often turns out to have been the MCT diet. We have found some children who continued to have seizures despite tolerating the MCT diet, but who subsequently responded well to the classic ketogenic diet. We have also seen many children and families who could not tolerate the MCT diet but who did well on the classic ketogenic diet. In other words, we at Hopkins have found that a little imagination applied to the classic ketogenic diet is more effective and more palatable than is the MCT formulation.

THE KETOGENIC DIET TODAY

These days, information on the nutritional content of almost all food is readily available. Numerous books provide nutritional information for a wide variety of foods. Information on processed foods, if not shown on the label, is available from the manufacturer upon request. The importance of nutrition is appreciated more than ever, as demonstrated by the prevalence of nutrition-based treatment for high cholesterol, diabetes, and renal or heart disease. At the same time, research has shown that all the modern medication and technology currently available cannot control some 20 percent of children with epilepsy.

Even now, of course, the diet requires a lot of work on the part of the parents as well as the dietitians, especially during the first weeks. Success on the diet requires patience, persistence, care, and faith on the part of the whole team: the physician and the dietitian as well as the parents and children. But for the 50 percent of children with difficult-to-control seizures, whose seizures are lessened or controlled by the diet, for those who are able to think more clearly because they have fewer medication side effects, the reemergence of the ketogenic diet has provided a new and better life than was obtained on any of the new anticonvulsant medications.

SECTION II

PROCESS

CHAPTER FOUR

INITIATING THE KETOGENIC DIET

INITIATION: A PROCESS

Initiating the ketogenic diet is a process, not an event. The initiation process begins when a child is accepted into a ketogenic diet program. Before admission to the hospital, the child's EEGs and other medical records are sent to us and reviewed. The parents are asked to write a letter describing their child and their personal goals for the diet.

There have been no firm criteria for accepting or rejecting children for diet initiation at Johns Hopkins. In general, however:

- Most (but not all) children will have more than two seizures per week.

- Most children will have failed at least two anticonvulsants.

- Occasionally we will accept children whose seizures have been controlled but only at the expense of toxicity.

The parents' goals—if realistic—are often the determining factor in our acceptance. Even then many families are referred to a ketogenic diet program closer to their homes. Parents are also asked to keep a seizure calendar for the month before hospitalization, to watch the video "Introduction to the Ketogenic Diet," and to read this book. The child's primary care physician is sent information about the diet, along with recommendations for treatment of illness while on the diet.

Just before admission at Johns Hopkins (other centers may have slightly different practices), the child is given an outpatient evaluation and attends a lesson on the history of the diet, which includes an overview of the expected course of the hospitalization (see Appendix B, "Johns Hopkins Hospital Nursing Critical Pathways").

Starting the diet requires about four days of hospitalization, beginning with fasting and followed by the gradual introduction of the high-fat meals. During the initial phase of the diet, which lasts several weeks, the body becomes adjusted to the smaller portions and lower calorie levels of the diet and to digesting the larger quantities of fat. It requires several weeks for the body to "learn" to utilize the fat for energy and to recover its former level of energy. During this period, the family becomes accustomed to weighing and measuring all meals, and the child gradually becomes adjusted to the foods of the diet and to not eating other foods.

Once this transition has been accomplished, it is possible to assess how well the diet is working in controlling seizures. Then the "fine-tuning" phase of the diet begins. This involves adjusting the various components of the diet—calories, liquids, fats, recipes, ketogenic ratios, and so forth—to achieve the best level of ketosis for optimal seizure control.

Initiating the diet means not only changing the foods that are consumed but also changing attitudes toward food, changing attitudes toward mealtimes, and changing the parents', family members', and friends' attitudes toward eating. These changes cannot take place immediately, but they are essential for long-term success on the diet.

Each child is different, and each family has its own idiosyncrasies. Sometimes the number of calories the child requires is overestimated at the start. Sometimes a child refuses to eat the cream or becomes too constipated. Adjustments to the child's diet must then be made. It takes at least two weeks to see if a change is effective. Since only one change can be made at a time, it may take several months of fine-tuning to see how much benefit the diet will provide for that child.

This is why a family is asked to make a three-month commitment to trying the diet before coming into the hospital to initiate the fasting phase of the diet initiation. Eighty-three percent of families remain on the diet for at least three months. Every family is told that they may discontinue the diet any time they wish. However, since the initiation of the diet is so very labor-intensive for both the family and the ketogenic diet team, this investment of time, effort, and money is not worthwhile for anyone if the diet is not given a good trial.

It is very common for families to be beset by doubts as they embark on the ketogenic diet. To quote a few of the comments:

- "We'll never be able to eat as a family again. Sam will have to eat by himself in the kitchen so he won't see us eating pizza."

- "Phyllis is a picky eater and she hates eggs. I'll never get her to eat every bite."

- "We both work, and then there are the other two. Where will we ever find time to weigh and measure the meals?"

- "Are we facing two years without a vacation or a restaurant meal?"

Time and again families have found ways to cope with their problems and concerns. They have concluded that all the hassle is more than worthwhile:

- **If** the diet is of sufficient benefit to the child

- **If** it helps to control the seizures

- **If** the child's medications can be reduced

- **If** behavioral side effects of the seizures or medications can be minimized

A team effort is needed to keep the child and the family on track and help them to get through this difficult start-up period. In addition to the parents, child, and family, the ketoteam at Hopkins includes a physician, dietitian, nurse, and counselor who are familiar with the diet. Because each plays an important role in both initiating and maintaining the diet, we have written this chapter from the perspective of each of these key parties.

GETTING READY FOR THE DIET: THE PARENTS' PERSPECTIVE

Psychological Preparation

The most important factor contributing to the success of the diet is the psychological factor. It requires a great deal of faith. The parents must *believe* that the diet can work. It requires a determination to get a child out of that medication haze, to stop those frustrating absence seizures, and to throw away the helmet that had to be worn as protection against head drop seizures.

Parents who start out as doubters will focus on the inevitable initial difficulties of the diet instead of focusing on the decrease in seizures and improved behavior of the child as the diet starts. Without faith, it will be too frustrating when the child accidentally uses the wrong toothpaste, when she is irritable and demanding, or when she gets sick and has a seizure three weeks into the treatment. It will be too sad if the child cries for afternoon cookies or Sunday night pizza.

If parents start out thinking positively, saying, "We will do whatever is necessary to give this diet a chance to work; the sacrifice is worthwhile if our child has a chance to become seizure-free," they are already halfway there. Most children will have fewer seizures and/or less medicine on the diet. The question will become whether the improvement is sufficient to continue the diet. Families will have a greater chance of success if they think of the opportunity to try the diet as a gift to the child, not as a punishment for having seizures.

Sometimes problems with the diet may not come from the parents. They may come from a "How-will-my-grandchild-know-it's-me-if-I-don't-bring-Hershey's-Kisses?" grandma, or from a jealous "How-come-Peter-gets-all-the-attention?" sister. The optimism and faith that will carry a family through the diet (pardon us if this sounds a bit preachy) has to come from a team effort, encompassing the whole family, especially the child. Once the diet is effective and the seizures are under better control, once the child is functioning better, it becomes much easier to maintain the momentum. At the start it can be very tough. It is the willingness of the parents to meet the challenge that will carry the family through.

> *AT FIRST YOU'RE GOING TO BE AFRAID OF TEMPTATION. You're going to feel bad about your child seeing others eat food he can't have. You'll be worried about what the diet's emotional effects will be. And you're going to be worried about whether your kid will cooperate. But you can live through it!*
>
> *If you have other kids, they can eat other foods. Try to be positive. The main thing to remember is, if the diet works your kid will be so happy to feel well again!* —CC

Statement of Expectations

It is helpful for each parent, independently, to write a paragraph outlining what he or she would consider "success" on the diet—for their child. At Johns Hopkins we require that each parent write such a statement and send it to us before the hospital admission.

- For some, success would be if the child's seizures were reduced by half.

- Others demand complete seizure control.

- Some say, "If we could only decrease or eliminate the medication, then we could see what she is really like. We can live with the seizures, it is the medication which is so difficult."

This statement of expectations forces parents to confront the question of what they expect of the diet. It frequently offers substantial insight into their hopes, strengths, desires, and ability to confront reality.

The statement can open the opportunity for a physician to discuss misunderstandings about the diet or misperceptions about a child's potential abilities. Parents often hope that the child's problems are *all* due to the medications, or *only* due to the seizures, and that the diet will miraculously make their child like one who was never ill. The written statement of expectations clarifies their beliefs. Filed in the child's medical chart, the statement offers a benchmark against which to assess progress when the child returns for follow-up.

Getting the Child's Cooperation

The diet is more likely to go smoothly if children are *enlisted*—rather than *ordered*—to participate in the diet. Children do not like having seizures. They do not like being different from their friends. Often, most of all, they do not like taking medications. They want to be cured of their seizures. If possible, explain to a child, in an age-appropriate fashion, how the diet may help fix these problems. If parents communicate their own enthusiasm for the diet as something worth trying, something that really might work, most children will buy in. They will feed on your enthusiasm. So don't start the diet if you and your child are not enthusiastic about trying it—without that enthusiasm, it will be too hard.

But no one should make promises that cannot be kept! Parents cannot guarantee to the child that the seizures will disappear completely or that there will be no more medication. These are *goals,* but they cannot be *promises.* Sticking to the diet will ultimately be the child's responsibility. Parents can help by giving children the psychological and emotional power to handle the tough parts. Role-playing may be useful. Parents can try rehearsing what to say in difficult situations. For instance, a parent might pretend to be a teacher offering a cracker at snack time, and let a child practice saying, "That's not on my diet, thank you!" Or a parent might pretend to be a friend trying to swap a sandwich for cheesecake at lunch and teach the child responses such as, "No, I'm on a magic diet. I have to eat my own food." Children on the diet usually exhibit amazing self-control and willpower. They often handle the diet far better than their parents do—especially when they are doing well.

*SARAH WAS FIVE YEARS OLD AND HAD HAD A STROKE AT BIRTH. Her
one-sided seizures were hard to control. But before undergoing surgery,
her family decided to try the ketogenic diet. Sarah did very well, and
her seizures were better for a time, but ultimately she did not have good
enough seizure control. Surgery was scheduled. Sarah would say, "What
I dream about is having french fries again when I'm not on the diet any
more." So the night before surgery a nurse brought Sarah french fries.
Sarah's response was "I can't have these. I'm still on my special diet."—JF*

Older children who try the ketogenic diet often need someone on
whom they can vent their anger and frustrations. It is far better if this
can be someone other than their parents. For teens and preteens, it may
help to set up special telephone times when they can call and talk to
a counselor. This may start with a weekly call and then become less frequent. Through these calls children can report successes and discuss
problems, receive reinforcement, and hear stories about others who
went through the same thing.

One of our counselor's favorite lines, when things seem particularly
bleak and a child wants to quit the diet, is "Hey, it's up to you. No one is
making you stay on the diet. You are always free to choose to stop the
diet, to go back to having seizures and taking medicine. It's all up to
you." Putting the responsibility back on the child eliminates the parents
and counselor as bad guys and empowers the child to see the reality that
if the diet is indeed working, the choices are really very simple.

*I TOLD MICHAEL, "IT'S YOUR PROBLEM and you have to solve it. We
are here to help you, but most of the work is going to be yours. You're a big
guy, you can handle it." Michael was six, and he never cheated. Michael
continued to be a "special kid." He stuck with the diet and now has been
off the diet for several years. He still has a rare seizure but does well in
school and is a first rate basketball player.—EH*

Special Equipment

The most essential pieces of equipment for the ketogenic diet are a
gram scale and a kit to test ketones in the urine.

Gram Scales

The gram scale is the main calculating tool for the diet, so it is extremely important. Parents must either buy a gram scale or make sure that the hospital plans to supply one for the family to take home. At Johns Hopkins we make a gram scale available to parents at cost. Providing this service ensures that all parents get an accurate scale while saving them the time and effort of searching for one themselves. The scale

SCALES CAN BE OBTAINED through most office supply stores. Electronic digital scales, although slightly more expensive, are more accurate to the gram than manual scales. Examples of suitable scales include:

Pelouse Scale Company
2120 Greenwood St.
Evanston, IL 60201
Phone: 1-800-654-8330
Fax: 1-800-627-7330
E-mail: www.healthometer.com
Electronic postal scale, Model PS2R1-P. Electric or battery-operated (adapter not included). List price $160.00. Distributors: Office Max or Office Depot.

OHAUS Corporation
29 Hanover Road
Florham Park, NJ 07932
Phone: 1-800-672-7722
Fax: 973-593-0359
E-mail: www.ohaus.com
Portable electronic scale with one gram accuracy, Model LS200. Electric or battery-operated with AD adapter. List price $99.00.

should be accurate, should display weights in one-tenth gram increments, and should be portable.

TESTING FOR URINARY KETONES

Strips for testing ketone levels in the urine are commonly available in drugstores, often combined with glucose tests used by diabetic patients. Keto Diastix, manufactured by the Ames Company, is one such test strip. Children on the ketogenic diet test urine daily with these "ketostix."

TESTING FOR BLOOD IN THE URINE

Parents are instructed to test the urine weekly for blood, which may be an early sign of kidney stones. Hemoglobin (blood) in the urine may be tested using Bayer Multistix 10SG, which tests for several things including hemoglobin and ketones. Since these strips are expensive, we recommend using them only once each week. A positive test for hemoglobin does NOT necessarily mean there is blood in the urine. The test should be repeated on several different specimens and then confirmed by a physician before a parent should become concerned.

OPTIONAL EQUIPMENT THAT MAY BE USEFUL

Parents have found a variety of equipment helpful while their children are on the ketogenic diet. The following is a list gathered from many parents. It is meant as a source of ideas. All of this equipment is optional. Parents may buy these supplies if and as needed:

- large collection of small plastic storage containers (such as Tupperware or margarine tubs)
- bendable straws for drinking every drop
- sippy cups (have lids and do not spill) for smaller children
- screw-top plastic beverage containers
- small rubber spatulas to be used as plate-cleaners
- one-, two-, four-, and six-ounce plastic cups
- measuring cup marked with milliliters or a graduated cylinder for weighing and measuring

- 10 cc syringe
- six or more Pyrex custard dishes for microwave cooking and freezing meals
- popsicle molds
- six-inch nonstick skillet for sautéing individual portions with easy cleanup
- travel cooler and/or insulated bag (useful to take home eggnog from hospital)
- one or two small Thermoses for school and travel
- toothpicks for picking up morsels of food to make eating fun
- blender
- milkshake wand or small hand beater
- portable dual-burner electric camping stove for trips
- masking tape for labels
- microwave oven

To repeat, **it is not necessary to own a lot of equipment before starting the diet: the above is simply a sample list from various parents.** Parents will gain more insight as to what equipment they will need as well as specific brands of food that are acceptable during their in-hospital ketogenic diet education. The only supplies that are absolutely necessary before starting the diet are a scale that measures in grams (to weigh foods) and strips for testing ketone levels in urine, which may be purchased or obtained from the hospital.

Special Foods

HEAVY WHIPPING CREAM

The only essential food research parents need to do before starting the diet is to find out whether their neighborhood heavy cream supply is 36 percent fat, 40 percent fat, or somewhere in between. The fat content of heavy whipping cream varies from one location to another, but most heavy cream is 36 percent fat. The content of available cream will affect the calculation of the diet, so it is important to find out what is available in a given neighborhood and to tell the dietitian before the child's diet is calculated. **Make sure that there is no sugar added!** The label should read:

Whipping Cream   Grade A Ultra-Pasteurized Heavy
                                  Serving Size = 1 tablespoon or 15 cc
                                  Calories from fat = 50

If you have any doubts about the content of your local cream, call the dairy directly. Dairies are required by law to know the fat percentage of the cream they supply. Remember: labeling laws do not require companies to list anything less than 1 gram of carbohydrate, protein, or fat, although fractional grams can affect the ketogenic diet! Once you find an acceptable brand, stick with it. Some local dairies will help to ensure that your local store stocks large containers of heavy whipping cream. Call your local dairy if you have any questions.

OTHER FOODS AND FLAVORINGS

Many parents use flavorings to make the diet more fun for kids. These include (*starred items must be calculated into the child's diet):

- *Baking chocolate
- Fruit-flavored sugar-free, caffeine-free diet soda such as Faygo or Walmart Free & Clear
- *Pure* flavoring extracts: vanilla, almond, lemon, maple, coconut, chocolate. Make certain that they are pure. Pure flavorings may be ordered from Bickford Flavorings (216-531-6006, or 1-800-283-8322)
- *Sugar-free flavored gelatin such as D-Zerta, Jell-O, or Royal
- Non-stick spray such as Pam or Mazola No-stick for cooking
- Carbohydrate-free, calorie-free, sweeteners. Saccharin (1/4 grain tablets of pure saccharin) is best. Other sweeteners, such as Equal (the blue packets), Sweet'N Low (the pink packets), and NutraSweet contain carbohydrates that can upset ketosis.

This list, like the equipment list, is intended as a source of ideas, not a *must-buy-right-away* order. The rest of the diet ingredients should be pure, fresh, simple foods: lean meat, fish, or poultry, bacon, eggs, cheese, fruit, vegetables, butter, mayonnaise, and canola or olive oil.

READ THE LABEL!!! Manufacturers often change the formulations of their products without prior notice. Therefore each time you buy a processed food product, even if you have used it before, you must read the label very carefully. Remember that labeling laws do not require disclosure of contents less than 1 gram. Call the manufacturer if you have any questions.

BEWARE OF HIDDEN CARBOHYDRATES!!! Beware of any foods or medicines containing carbohydrates. Other nonsugar carbohydrates include those containing mannitol, sorbitol, dextrin, and many ingredients ending in "-ose," such as maltose, lactose, fructose, glucose, sucrose, dextrose, or polycose. All of these are carbohydrates and can be broken down into glucose. They either should not be used or must be calculated into the diet. Many foods, candies, and gums that are billed as "sugar-free" are NOT carbohydrate-free and cannot be used on the ketogenic diet.

BARBARA AND MICHELLE: TWO CARBOHYDRATE SAGAS

Barbara had had no seizures in six months and was doing superbly well on the ketogenic diet. In preparation for her follow-up EEG, the technician inadvertently gave her liquid chloral hydrate to allow her to sleep. But oral chloral hydrate is in a carbohydrate base. The technician should have used carbohydrate-free chloral hydrate suppositories instead. It does not take much carbohydrate to quickly negate ketosis. Barbara's first seizure in six months occurred during that EEG.

Michelle lived in the city, but during the summer the family spent weekends at their beach house. She did well on the diet throughout the winter, with a marked decrease in seizure frequency. In the summer she again began having increased seizures, although only on weekends.

The family would go to their summer house on Fridays. By Saturday Michelle's ketones would be low, and her seizures would increase. Her parents turned themselves inside out attempting to find the reason. They checked the foods, the environment, and finally decided she must be allergic to the beach and their pool. They were about to sell the house.

At last, together with a nurse from Johns Hopkins, they again went over everything they did on Friday and Saturday. "When we arrived at the beach, we lathered Michelle with suntan lotion," they told the nurse. Aha! They checked the suntan lotion label: it was in a sorbitol base. Apparently enough sorbitol was absorbed through Michelle's skin to affect her ketones and alter her seizure threshold! After switching to a sorbitol-free suntan lotion, the family continued taking Michelle to the beach with no recurrence of seizures.

Lowering ketosis through consumption of carbohydrates does not always cause such dramatic breakthrough seizures, but it can. The good news is that when isolated breakthrough seizures occur, they nearly always can be eliminated again once the source is traced.

Medications

Medications play an important role in the ultimate success of the ketogenic diet. Starches and sugars are frequently used as fillers and taste enhancers in all forms of medication—tablets, capsules, and particularly liquid medications. These starches and sugars can easily be overlooked in diet formulation, but they can impair a child's ability to maintain high levels of ketosis. **Read the labels of all medications carefully.** Take into account the carbohydrate content of all medications, whether routine medications taken daily or intermittent medications given to treat conditions such as a cold or an infection.

Ideally, the total carbohydrate content in medications should be less than 0.1 g (or 100 mg) for the entire day. Anything higher should be calculated into the meal plan's daily carbohydrate allotment. For example, a child taking 0.09 g (90 mg) of phenobarbital at bedtime in the form of three 0.03 g (30 mg) tablets receives 0.07 g (72 mg) of starch and lactose per tablet, or a daily total of 0.21 g (216 mg). There are carbohydrate-free forms of most of the older anticonvulsants. For example, Valproate in the sugar-free form of Sprinkles can be used. Some of the new anti-convulsants do not come in sugar-free form. If they must be continued, the carbohydrate content should be calculated into the diet. In some instances, the sugar-free intravenous form of the medication can be used orally. During the starvation and diet initiation phase of the diet, the carbohydrate content of medications should be minimized by avoiding liquid preparations. The filler in pills may be ignored or calculated into the carbohydrates allotted.

Difficulty in prescribing medications for a child on the ketogenic diet often arises from the fact that many common over-the-counter and prescription medications are not available in a sugar-free form. Many of those listed as "sugar-free" in references are appropriate for use in the diabetic population but not for children on the ketogenic diet because they contain starch or carbohydrates in the form of sugar substitutes such as sorbitol and mannitol.

The Food and Drug Administration does not require the listing of inactive ingredients such as sorbitol in the labeling of oral prescription drugs. Even when ingredients are listed, their precise amounts are often not found on the label.

Additionally, manufacturers frequently are reluctant to release information about the amounts of particular ingredients in a medication, contending that this is proprietary information or that formulations change frequently. However, they can usually be persuaded to release the information if it is for treatment of a specific patient.

A pharmacist who is willing to get to know the ketogenic diet and the child and to work with the family for the duration of the diet can be a valuable asset, helping to interpret labels and calling manufacturers if necessary. When starting the diet, locate a source of:

- sugar-free and lactose-free multivitamins, such as Mead Johnson's Poly-Vi-Sol (liquid or drops) with iron or Mead Johnson's Unicap-M

- carbohydrate-free calcium, such as Rugby's calcium gluconate (600 to 650 mg) or Calcimix (500 mg)

- carbohydrate-free toothpaste such as Tom's Natural, Arm & Hammer, or Ultra brite

Routine medications that are taken daily should come from a single company, as ingredient concentrations vary among manufacturers. General rules for the use of medications, a selected list of medications that have been used by children on the diet, and contact information for pharmaceutical manufacturers can be found in Appendix A at the back of this book. Most medications can also be made in a carbohydrate-free form by a compounding pharmacy. You can ask a local one or order from Ridge Pharmacy (1-800-RIDGE-RX).

STARTING ON THE KETOGENIC DIET

The Ketogenic Diet Team

The ketogenic diet is always a team effort. The size of the team will depend on the institution. The team always involves a physician and a dietitian knowledgeable about the diet. The dietitian must allocate the time not only to teach the diet while the family is in the hospital for diet initiation but also to help the family with questions and dietary changes after discharge. Some medical centers also have a nurse or physician's assistant who can help the family through the many small crises that do not require medical attention. At Johns Hopkins we also assign each new family a "ketocoach," a parent who has been through the diet successfully, to provide additional nonmedical support.

RACHEL WAS STARTED ON THE DIET at a major children's hospital. The dietitian there was very nice, but very busy since she had to cover the whole hospital. The diet worked well in the hospital, but a week after Rachel went home, her seizures began increasing. Her mother checked everything, then called the hospital. The dietitian said that she couldn't help with fine-tuning because she only worked with children in the hospital, not with outpatients. Rachel's mother was outraged!

If a center is going to start children on the diet, it must also be prepared to adjust the diet and work with the family for at least several months after discharge. The successful management of difficult-to-control seizure patients and the fine-tuning of the diet are labor-intensive and time-consuming. **We estimate that an average family requires 40 telephone hours of dietary and illness counseling during the first year on the diet.**

Preparing for Admission

We find that it is easier to admit three or four patients simultaneously for the ketogenic diet than to do it one at a time. The advantage of admitting several patients at once is not only the efficiency of teaching the daily classes to multiple individuals but also the support that families in the group can provide to each other as they go through the learning curve and the tribulations of diet initiation together. Without the group there is a tendency for each parent to feel that he or she is the only person in the whole world who is burdened with such an overwhelming task. Families in each group often stay in contact after hospital discharge and are brought back for follow-up on the same day.

Groups are usually admitted every two weeks, which allows us to get one group off to a good start before the next one comes in. When we accept a child specifically for our fine-tuning program, that child can be scheduled at the same time.

The inpatient hospital stay is four days, with an outpatient visit and a teaching session on the day before admission. People often ask why a child has to be hospitalized while starting the diet. The reasons are that in a hospital:

- Physicians can supervise the fasting and guard against potentially serious symptoms of hypoglycemia, dehydration, or severe acidosis.

- Physicians can, if necessary, adjust medication levels according to the child's needs. Although medication should not be reduced more than necessary for several weeks, until the child and family adjust to the diet, it often is necessary to

EXCESS KETOACIDOSIS   occurs with 15 percent to 20 percent of our
children starting the diet and may require either IV fluids or fluids
given by a nasogastric tube for the first several days.

eliminate or sharply reduce phenobarbital and acetazo-
lamide (Diamox) to prevent toxicity and too much sleepiness
during the fasting and early acidosis.

• The ketoteam can meet intensively with parents and train
them to prepare the diet and deal with common physical and
psychosocial issues that may arise.

*Robert was a frail three-year-old with very difficult to control
"drop" spells. His mother was eager to get started on the diet, and eliminated all starches and carbohydrates three days before coming to Hopkins.*

*The fasting was started, and the next morning Robert was admitted
to the hospital. That night he vomited once and did not want to take his
fluids. The next morning he was very sleepy. By that evening he had
vomited twice and vomited his first eggnog.*

*Blood tests showed that Robert was too ketotic, and without enough
fluids he was also somewhat dehydrated. Some fluids and a small amount
of glucose put him back on track and allowed him to take the eggnog and
progress to the diet.*

CHAPTER FIVE

FINE-TUNING THE DIET: THE KEY TO SUCCESS

GOALS OF THE FINE-TUNING PROCESS

Fine-tuning the ketogenic diet involves the manipulation of a child's calories and ketogenic ratio, meal plans, eating patterns, liquid allotments, and other variables in order to achieve optimal seizure control. The first few weeks after a child's discharge from the hospital is often the most intensive fine-tuning period. This initial period of fine-tuning is, we believe, the key to long-term success or failure on the ketogenic diet.

We encourage close telephone communication with the ketoteam during the first few weeks that a child is on the ketogenic diet. This support can be crucial as the family becomes accustomed to preparing the diet and integrates it into their lifestyle. Myriad questions arise as the diet is initiated and as the meals are prepared. Support for fine-tuning is particularly necessary when seizure control improves initially but the family is hoping for even better seizure control or for the child to be on even less medication.

> **THE GOALS OF FINE-TUNING THE DIET ARE:**
> 1. To reduce seizures to a minimum—optimally for the child to become free of seizures.
> 2. To reduce seizure medications to a minimum—optimally for the child to become free of anticonvulsant medications.

EXPECTATIONS

Fine-tuning does not always lead to total freedom from seizures. During the initiation of the ketogenic diet and afterward, it helps if a family's expectations are realistic, so that they are not setting themselves up for disappointment. Virtually all families have watched the videotape from the Charlie Foundation before diet initiation. In this tape it appears that Charlie Abrahams came to Hopkins severely impaired by his seizures and medications and walked out of the hospital four days later cured. This impression is reinforced by the story of the child with uncontrollable seizures in the Meryl Streep film *First Do No Harm*. That child was also flown to Johns Hopkins and sent home cured.

These stories are both based on truth, but they are not typical, and certainly not universal:

- Not everyone is cured by the ketogenic diet.
- Not all of those whose seizures are substantially helped by the diet find the correct calorie level and ketogenic ratio during their initial stay in the hospital.
- Not all children are able to come off medication and remain seizure-free.

With careful fine-tuning, however, more than one-half of the children starting the ketogenic diet at Johns Hopkins derive sufficient benefit that they remain on the diet for more than one year.

Even Charlie Abrahams required a fine-tuning period. Charlie didn't go home from the hospital in four days. He remained several extra days in the hospital, sick and vomiting, until it was determined a virus was causing his nausea. Even after he had returned home, it took days for Charlie to feel well. After this initial difficult time, Charlie became seizure-free and eventually medication-free. Still, he was often reluctant to eat, and persuading him to finish each meal was a major daily struggle for his mother. Two years later, when coming off the diet, he again had several seizures. Now, five years later, Charlie remains on a modified version of the ketogenic diet.

The lessons to be learned from Charlie's case are important. Charlie's experience with the diet was, and is, a spectacular success. But this success did not come easily. When obstacles arose, his parents refused to become disappointed and discouraged. They put in a lot of hard work, maintained a tough attitude, and made the diet work for Charlie.

The most important thing for a parent to remember during the fine-tuning period is: **you can, and you must, persevere!** If your child is doing well at the start of the diet, terrific! But most children do not immediately become seizure-free. Many never become totally free of seizures; others do become virtually, or even totally, seizure-free after weeks or months of careful fine-tuning.

Only after working carefully with the ketoteam for several months will you have enough information to decide if there is sufficient improvement in your child to continue with the diet.

If seizures are controlled for even a few days at the start, the diet is likely to work. Long-term control can likely be established with patient fine-tuning. We suspect that at the end of two days of fasting and the two days of gradual introduction of the ketogenic eggnog, a child's blood serum ketones may reach a peak, providing a temporarily high level of seizure control. Once the child is at home and eating meals again, serum ketones may not be as high, even though the urine is still 4+. Increasing the ketosis by fine-tuning the diet may help.

Breakthrough seizures do not necessarily mean that the diet has failed; further fine-tuning is likely to be beneficial. If seizures are improved, less frequent, or less severe, it may be hoped that further improvement will be achieved as the diet is adjusted.

Some of the factors that may have to be adjusted during this fine-tuning period are calorie allotment and distribution, the ketogenic ratio, meal plans, meal frequency, liquid intake, fiber content, and anticonvulsant medication levels.

THE IMPORTANCE OF SLEUTHING

To master the fine-tuning process, parents and the ketoteam become adept at tracing the cause of any problem that arises. If a child is having problems on the diet, the parents and the rest of the diet team must become private eyes. It often takes a detective's spirit to locate the source of a problem and fix it. The most common cause of a problem with the diet is that the child is getting the wrong amount or the wrong balance of food and liquid. There could be many reasons why the amount or balance of food and liquid are off:

- Is there an opportunity for the child to eat extra food at school or while playing at a friend's house?
- Is the diet prescription correctly calculated? The caloric needs of a disabled child may be much lower than those of a non-handicapped child of the same age and size.
- Are commercial foods being used?
- If commercial foods are used, are they the exact brands and items called for in the menu?
- Check the label—has the manufacturer changed ingredients?
- If calculations were made by computer, are the database entries for the ingredients correct?
- Is the child gaining weight?
- Is the child sick with a common virus or bacterial infection?
- Is everything being measured on a gram scale except free fluids?

- Are Group B vegetables being measured properly, differently from Group A vegetables?
- Are vegetables being weighed cooked or raw as specified?
- Are the peaches packed in water, as they should be, rather than in glucose-containing syrup or fruit juice?
- Is there a soft-hearted grandparent in the picture who is encouraging the child to cheat "just a little?"

It is not possible to list every problem and solution in this book, but the principle to remember is: be a sleuth. Think it through. Don't give up. Look for clues. Was there a change in the number or kind of seizures at a certain time of the day or week? Problems following a certain meal plan or a specific family event?

JESSICA CAME IN FOR A CHECKUP after a year on the diet and she was doing great. She talked like a little adult, whereas before the diet she had difficulty making sentences at all because her mind was so full of seizures. She was still having some seizures, though. What she told us was that her grandmother liked to give her candy even though the candy gave her seizures. She said she was going to change that, though. She was going to start saying, "I can't have any more candy, Grandma. I'm on a special diet and I have to stay on my diet because I don't like having seizures!" Jessica had to stay on the diet for longer than the usual period of time. She would probably have gotten off sooner if her grandmother hadn't cheated. —MK

If a problem develops after good seizure control has been established, parents should examine every aspect of their child's food and liquid intake, play habits, pharmaceuticals, and time with babysitters and relatives. The dietitian should listen to a parent describing exactly how each meal is prepared. If the dietitian cannot solve the problem, the physician may need to get involved. With persistence you can most likely isolate the problem and correct it.

Remember: Illness, ear infection, the flu, or urinary tract infection may also cause breakthrough seizures. See if your child is sick before you change the diet.

MEASURING KETOSIS

The efficacy of fine-tuning is measured by a child's seizure control, but also by her level of ketosis. It is presumed that the ketogenic diet produces seizure control by changing the brain's metabolism to one based on ketones rather than carbohydrate. This is achieved by dramatically reducing the child's carbohydrate intake and eating a diet high in fat. The incompletely metabolized fat leaves residual ketone bodies, which the brain then uses as its energy source (see Chapter 1). The specific goal of fine-tuning, then, is to get the brain into a state of ketosis adequate to obtain optimal seizure control.

We teach parents to check daily ketones by using a urine dipstick. This is an easy, cost-effective method for monitoring the level of ketosis. The paper stick, when dipped in the child's urine, turns color depending on the amount of ketones in the urine. The ketogenic diet has traditionally been fine-tuned to maintain the child's urine at 3–4+ ketones, which turn the stick a dark purple in color (80–160 mmol).

For babies and young children who are not yet toilet-trained, urine is collected by placing cotton balls in the diaper. Once the child has urinated, the cotton balls can be squeezed onto a dipstick for testing. For older children on the diet, peeing on a dipstick becomes second nature.

The weakness of urinary ketone testing is that it is actually ketones in the brain, not those in the urine, that influence seizure control. Ketones in the urine can seem lower if tested after a child drinks a large quantity of liquid. They may vary with the time of day. These ups and downs, however, may have only an indirect relation to seizure control.

We predict that measuring ketones in the blood may provide a more accurate picture of ketosis relevant to seizure control. Technology is now in development that will allow the measurement of ketones in the blood on a finger prick of blood, just as diabetics currently measure their own blood sugar. When blood (serum) ketone tests at home are commercially available, the goal of "fine-tuning" the diet may become to produce certain levels of blood ketones rather than testing the amount which spills out in the urine. However, until serum ketone tests are readily and inexpensively available, urinary assessment remains the best (and only) available tool to monitor a child's ketosis.

Preliminary evidence using blood ketones suggests that once the blood ketone level rises to more than 2 mmol, the urine ketone level becomes 4+. That is the highest level the dipstix can measure. Seizure control however, appears far better when serum levels are greater than 4 mmol, way beyond that 4+ urine level. So, a urine ketone test of 4+ is **necessary** to establish that the child has ketosis but **not sufficient** to indicate very good ketosis. It is to be hoped that serum ketone tests may permit a level of seizure control beyond what is now possible.

COMMON PROBLEMS AT THE START OF THE DIET

Two to three weeks after the hospital discharge, the child and the family will have had the chance to adapt to the diet as it was initially calculated (for principles of diet calculation, see Chapter 8). This is the time we start making the small changes we call "fine-tuning," that can often make a major difference in a child's level of seizure control. The most common areas to be explored for fine-tuning potential are:

- Caloric intake
- Carbohydrate intake
- Distribution of meals
- Misuse of free foods
- Menu preparation
- Illness
- Ketogenic ratio
- Fluid intake
- Processed food content
- Function or use of gram scales
- Food values used in calculations

Nearly every child whose seizures are somewhat, but not entirely, controlled on the diet two to three weeks after discharge will benefit, to some degree, from a period of fine-tuning.

Weight Gain

The most common error in initiating the diet is the improper estimation of a child's caloric needs. For some children the initial estimate of calories and ratio is appropriate, or at least sufficient, and seizures are completely controlled on the diet as initially prescribed. For some children, however, overestimation of caloric needs means that while seizures decrease after the initiation process, they are not as well controlled as they could be.

Overestimation of calories takes place partly because the recommended daily allowances (RDAs) of calories on which diet calculations are based are for average children of a given height and weight, with an average level of activity. (See Chapter 8, "Calculating the Ketogenic Diet," for more details.) However, the ketogenic diet is often used with children whose motor capabilities are impaired to the point that they burn far fewer calories than average, healthy children.

TAMMY, A SEVERELY DAMAGED 9-MONTH-OLD, was very inactive. Her only activity, in fact, was multiple flexion seizures, more than 100 per day. Her height was at only the 5th percentile, but her weight, at 24 pounds, was at the 90th percentile, possibly as the result of steroids used to treat her seizures. In order to get her into ketosis adequate for seizure control, she needed to be brought down closer to her desirable weight.

The ketogenic diet calculation for Tammy was set according to her basal calorie level (that needed just to maintain bodily function), 428 calories/day, about half that of an average, active 9-month-old. After 15 months on the ketogenic diet, Tammy weighed 21.5 pounds, so that her height and weight were both at the 5th percentile.

As she approached her desirable weight and had less body fat to burn to make ketones, Tammy's ketone levels began to drop and the ketogenic ratio was raised to 4:1. By the time she was two years old, Tammy's seizures had decreased more than 95 percent. She had seizures only rarely, during illness.

It is tempting to start small, profoundly handicapped children on calories that are geared to more active children of the same height and weight, as a dietitian will usually prefer to err on the high side than to underestimate calories. However, we often find that such children gain weight at this calorie level, and it becomes necessary to cut back. It may be preferable to take better account of the child's activity level when making the original calculations. Restricting calories for less active children will result in better ketosis and earlier improvement in seizure control. It is also psychologically easier for families to add calories or a snack to the diet than to reduce calories.

Weight Loss

If a child has lost a pound in one month, calculation will reveal that approximately 100 calories should be added to the daily diet. With these additional calories, the child should gain back the lost pound in a month. Once the child's proper caloric intake is reached, the weight gain or loss will stop. Remember: no two children are identical. Basal metabolic rates differ from child to child, and activity levels can differ markedly. In each case, excessive weight gain or loss indicates that caloric intake must be adjusted.

If a child is losing too much weight, the calorie level should be increased in increments of approximately 100 calories at a time. When

TO GREATLY OVERSIMPLIFY, for average people it takes approximately 3,500 calories to gain a pound. If a child has gained a pound in one month, then 3,500 too many calories have been consumed. Dividing the calories by the number of days (31 in a typical month) reveals that the child has consumed approximately 100 extra calories each day. By recalculating the diet at about 100 fewer calories, the dietitian can stop the weight gain.

THE HUNGER PARADOX Ketosis is an appetite suppressant. If reducing calories on the diet leads to better ketosis, it may decrease hunger as well. Therefore, children who are getting too many calories and gaining weight on the diet may feel hungrier than those who are getting fewer calories. Children who are hungry on he diet may have been given too much to eat! There-fore, *reducing calories may relieve hunger.*

increasing calories in infants or very inactive children, it is best to increase by 25 calories every 1 to 2 weeks until you reach the desired caloric level, since too rapid an increase seems to precipitate seizures.

Enough time should pass between increments so that an evaluation can be made as to whether the child's weight has stabilized, whether seizure activity has occurred or increased, and whether hunger is under control. If it is determined that extra calories are needed, instead of recalculating all the meal plans, a snack calculated at the prescribed ratio of fat to carbohydrate and protein may be added to the diet (calculating calories and ratios is further explained in Chapter 8). Adding a ketogenic eggnog snack to the child's daily meal plan may be a convenient alternative to recalculating all the meals in the short term while adjustments to the diet are being made. Twelve grams of macadamia nuts, which equals 100 calories, also make a good snack (the macadamia nuts, naturally in a 3:1 ratio, are sometimes eaten with a calculated amount of butter to achieve a 4:1 ratio).

Hunger

Because the physical quantity of food on the diet (the bulk) is smaller than in a normal diet, many children will feel hungry during the first week or two of the diet until they adjust. This may be especially true of overweight children, who will have their diets calculated to include some weight loss. However, ketosis itself decreases the appetite, so children are much less likely to be hungry when consistently high levels of ketones are reached, usually within a week of starting the diet.

If a child initially complains of being hungry, try to determine whether:

- she is really hungry
- she has not yet adapted to the smaller portion
- what she wants is the pleasure and comfort of eating

Sometimes it is not the child who is hungry at all, but rather the parents who feel pity for the child or guilt about the small portions, and who project their feelings about the diet onto the child. Other times, in the complex emotional atmosphere of diet initiation, a child's cries of hunger are actually declarations of rebellion against the parents. In any case, most children will lose their feelings of hunger once they adjust to the food they are consuming and achieve consistently high ketosis.

We recommend that parents deal with hunger without trying to add extra calories to the diet, at least for the first few weeks. Tricks to modify hunger without increasing calories include:

- drinking decaffeinated diet soda or seltzer instead of water for at least part of the liquid allotment
- freezing drinks, such as diet orange soda mixed with cream, into popsicles
- eating a leaf of lettuce twice a day with meals
- eating Group A vegetables or 10 percent fruits, since greater quantities of these are allowed
- making sure that foods such as vegetables are patted dry so that water is not part of the weight
- recalculating the diet plan into four equal meals, or three meals and a snack, while maintaining a constant level of calories and the proper ketogenic ratio
- decreasing calories slightly to raise ketosis and suppress hunger

CELESTE, AGE 2, HAD BEEN HOME FROM THE HOSPITAL *four days when her father called the doctor. "My wife is exhausted from staying with*

Celeste in the hospital," he said. "Now Celeste won't eat anything. She's crying, she's sleepy, she's whining all the time. We can't live like this!" His voice cracked with exasperation. "I can't take this diet!"

"How many seizures was she having last week, before she went into the hospital?" the doctor asked.

"More than a hundred every day."

"How many did she have during the starvation?"

"About ten a day."

"How many did she have yesterday at home?"

"One!"

"Let's not give up the on diet so fast then," the doctor replied. "Maybe there's a reason why she is so sleepy and irritable."

On further investigation, it was discovered that Celeste had developed a fever, and her pediatrician diagnosed a urinary tract infection. Once this was treated, Celeste continued on the diet and did very well.

Non-Diet Problems

When problems appear in a child on the ketogenic diet, don't always assume that the diet is the cause of the problem. A child may be irritable from the hospital stay or from the difficulty of making such a radical adjustment in her life. She may rebel against the extra attention and pressure to which she is being exposed. She may be coming down with the flu or a cold like any other child. A cautious approach to fine-tuning over several weeks or months after diet initiation will allow parents and the ketoteam to separate diet-related problems from other factors in the child's life.

THIRST

Liquid levels in the ketogenic diet are usually set at around 60 cc per kilogram of body weight or approximately one cc per calorie on the diet. One of the goals of the diet is to maintain the body in a minimally hydrated state. Liquid levels must strike a balance between being high enough for adequate body function without being so high that they adversely affect the diet. Too little liquid càn result in kidney stones (see section below).

It seems to be important for many children to space the consumption of liquids throughout the day and not to give a thirsty child a big drink all at once, as this can sometimes cause breakthrough seizure activity and can also leave the child more thirsty later on. Some parents give their children a regular dose of water or diet soda (with no caffeine) every one to two hours during the day. Other children seem to be able to drink larger amounts of liquid with no seizures.

In hot climates or during summer months, the cream in the diet need not be counted as part of the allotted liquid. In effect, this raises the liquid allowance by the quantity of the cream.

A child may become dehydrated if the fluid allowance is insufficient. Signs of dehydration include dry lips and skin, infrequent urination, sunken eyes, and lethargy. Most thirst problems, as well as problems of excessive acidosis, can be corrected by increasing fluid intake, usually in increments of 10 to 20 cc/kg of body weight per day until the problem is corrected. The ketoteam can determine adequate fluid replacement levels and ongoing fluid requirements by monitoring a child's weight, urine quantity, specific gravity of the urine, and ketone levels.

Kidney Stones

Painful renal stones occur in as many as one in six children on the ketogenic diet, probably as a result of inadequate fluid intake. To help children avoid developing kidney stones, parents test urine once a week with a "Hematest" dipstick for specific gravity and blood.

If blood is detected in the urine, a child is instructed to drink freely for 48 hours, following which the fluid allotment is increased. If blood in the urine persists despite this increase in fluid, a urine sample is sent to a lab, where tests for calcium, creatinine, and uric acid levels, as well as reagent strip analysis and microanalysis are conducted.

A renal sonogram may be necessary if the calcium to creatinine ratio is above 0.2 mg and/or the urine remains positive for blood. The child is started on Bicitra or Polycitra K to alkalinize the urine and dissolve the crystals. With alkalinization even established stones may disappear. If stones do not resolve with this treatment, lithotripsy or, on rare occasions, even surgical removal of kidney stones may be necessary.

Other signs of possible kidney stones include sharp abdominal pain and nonspecific illness with fever, poor appetite, or an unexplained increase in seizures.

SLEEPINESS AND SEDATION

On the ketogenic diet, excess sleepiness or lethargy can be due to excessive ketosis or toxicity. Medication levels frequently rise in the blood of children on the ketogenic diet even without a change in dosage. Medication levels may rise due to the partial dehydration state, altered serum binding, elevated drug levels in the brain, or changes in drug metabolism. Medication levels should be monitored carefully during the fasting and diet initiation period, and those medications that cause drowsiness, such as phenobarbital and benzodiazepines, should be decreased if sleepiness occurs.

Some children on the diet have lab results showing medications at therapeutic levels but exhibit signs of medication toxicity that improve when the drug dose is lowered. Although fasting and diet initiation can cause lethargy, the symptoms should rarely persist beyond 2 to 3 weeks.

Some children become more alert and energetic while on the ketogenic diet. This may be a result of taking fewer medications or having fewer seizures. As mentioned in Chapter 5, hypoglycemia or low blood sugar levels can also cause lethargy during the initial fasting period, but blood sugar levels should return to normal within a few days of starting the diet.

CONSTIPATION

Constipation can become a problem because of the small volume of food, low fiber content, reduced fluid intake, and high concentration of fat in this diet. Constipation may cause stomach pains and discomfort. Fortunately, it does not have to be an obstacle to continuing the diet. Using Group A vegetables in meal plans can help increase the bulk and fiber in the diet a little bit. Also, two leaves of lettuce, or about one-half cup of chopped lettuce, are allowed each day as so-called "free" food.

Make sure that the child is receiving the proper amount of liquid. Increasing daily liquid levels by 100 to 150 cc may help combat constipation.

If a child continues to have problems with constipation, laxatives, stool softeners, or enemas may help. Full-strength enemas should not be used regularly because they can affect the lining of the intestine. Small amounts of Colace (1% solution or suppository), Milk of Magnesia, Epsom salts, or MCT oil calculated into the diet might be effective in maintaining bowel regularity and preventing constipation. All laxatives must be sugar-free.

FINE-TUNING MEAL PLANS

As mentioned in Chapter 4, each child is given several (about six) meal plans, calculated by the dietitian specifically for that child, before leaving the hospital at diet initiation. These meal plans will probably be in the form of "chicken (or meat, or egg), Group B vegetable (or 10% fruit), fat, cream." As the child adjusts to the diet, the meal plans themselves may need fine-tuning. Physical reasons, such as weight loss or weight gain, may necessitate revising the meal plans, or a child may refuse to eat a basic diet component such as cream.

As parents prepare the diet meal, they will learn from their children what works and what does not work for them. The child who loves chocolate cream popsicles, for instance, may want to eat chocolate cream popsicles at every lunch and dinner. The child who leaves the hospital with six basic meal plans may grow tired of them after a period and want more variety.

Once parents get the hang of using their gram scales and making up specific menus, some want to devise their own menus or add little treats to the diet to increase the child's enjoyment of meals or ability to participate in family events. Adding or changing ingredients is limited only by the mathematical confines of the ketogenic ratio and by the child's protein requirement.

A computer program can help parents to devise meal plans that incorporate specific foods a child likes. One such software program is

NO MEALS SHOULD BE CREATED by parents until-fine tuning has been accomplished. Adding "fancy foods" just adds to the difficulty of teasing out what is wrong when ketones are low.

available from the Johns Hopkins Pediatric Epilepsy Center; the address can be found at the front of this book.

Of course, fats, carbohydrates, and protein must be kept in proper balance, and enough protein must be supplied in the diet to support a child's physical development. Still, parents and dietitians can find ways to include treats for the children that are properly calculated into the diet. After all, the object of the ketogenic diet is to control seizures. Within the limits of this goal, the diet can be made as easy as possible for a child to live with.

Parents should carefully research any and all new foods they wish to introduce into the diet, especially commercially processed foods. Foods whose protein, fat, and carbohydrate content are not clearly labeled should be avoided. So-called diet foods or sugar-free foods such as chewing gum may contain carbohydrates that make them inappropriate for the diet or at least makes it necessary that they be calculated in. This topic is addressed more thoroughly in Chapters 4 and 7.

"Free" Foods

There are no foods on the ketogenic diet that are actually "free," meaning available on an unlimited basis. What are often referred to as "free" foods are those that can be eaten occasionally in small quantities without being calculated into the daily ketogenic menu plans.

Free foods include 25 grams of lettuce; one walnut, macadamia nut, or pecan; three filberts; or three ripe (black) olives. Most other foods, such as sugar-free Jell-O or any carbohydrate-based snack food, cannot be used at all without being calculated into the diet.

Any added foods outside of meal plans can make a difference in seizure control. Children who eat free foods every day may find that they affect seizure control. For children who continue to have seizures on the diet, free foods should be the first thing restricted during the fine-tuning process.

> **WHEN SHE CAME TO US,** *Jennifer was tied in a wheelchair. She was so impaired by her drop seizures and her medications that she couldn't stand. She was already on a low-protein diet because her liver had been damaged by medication. Five days after she started the initial fast and ketogenic diet she was running down the hall! Everybody was so excited. Back home, she didn't need naps anymore. Her anticonvulsants were stopped. She was doing so well and not having any seizures. Then the seizures came back, a little bit at first, and of course we had to recheck everything. It turned out that Jennifer liked nuts. She was allowed two "free" nuts per day. But her mother had started giving her extra nuts, seven per day, because she was begging for them and they made her so happy. When we went back to two nuts a day the seizures came back under control.—MK*

Specific Foods

Initial menus for the diet are usually calculated using "generic" fruits and vegetables but designating specific meats and fats. Vegetables are placed in Group A or Group B, depending on their carbohydrate content. Group A vegetables have less carbohydrate, so the quantity of Group A vegetables in a given menu can be twice the amount of Group B vegetables. Within the generic groups, foods are interchangeable. This approach is easier for families and allows parents to pick from a list of varied fruits and vegetables.

However, the foods within these lists actually vary in content, and that variation can affect optimal seizure control for some patients. For example, 10 percent (Group B) fruits actually vary in carbohydrate content from 7 grams per 100 grams (strawberries) to over 17 grams per 100 grams (purple grapes).

Fresh meats vary even more widely. One hundred grams of lean ground beef contains 24 grams of protein, while 100 grams of pork chop contains 32 grams of protein. One hundred grams of eye round beef contains only 6.5 grams of fat, while 100 grams of lean ground beef contains about 19 grams of fat. For this reason, meats are not given in the form of a generic exchange list.

For many children this level of variation is unimportant, but for some children it appears to make the difference between inadequate ketosis to control seizures and sufficient ketosis. Therefore, when a child needs fine-tuning we try calculating the menus with exact foods instead of using generic food groups. Using the computer to calculate individual diets with specific foods can make a large difference in ketosis and therefore in seizure control.

The use of processed foods such as hot dogs and deli meats may cause a drop in urine ketones and result in a rise of seizures. The content of these foods is hard to assess. The labeling of their content is not exact. They are usually high in carbohydrates and sodium and relatively low in protein. These issues make them not only poor choices for maintaining optimum ketones but also poor for supplying adequate protein. Therefore, while fine-tuning the diet of a child with continued seizure activity, parents are requested to withhold processed foods for one month to see if this has an effect.

Fats

Not all fats are equal. A child who is having difficulty producing sufficient ketosis may need to have the *type* of fats in her diet adjusted. It may help to reduce or remove the less dense fats such as butter and mayonnaise and substitute canola, flaxseed, olive, or MCT oil (Table 5-1). Medium-chain triglyceride (MCT) oil is more efficiently metabolized, helping to produce a deeper ketosis. We use MCT oil for only a portion of the fat allowance, however, because when ingested in large quantities, it often causes gastrointestinal disturbances such as diarrhea or vomiting.

At Johns Hopkins we suggest using, as much as possible, unsaturated oils that contain a high fat level per gram and little or no carbohydrate or protein. Flaxseed oil is a good, heart-healthy choice. When using MCT oil, we begin with 5 grams per meal, or 15 total grams daily, for children who need to go into deeper ketosis. This may be increased slowly, as tolerated, until seizure control seems as good as possible with minimal side effects.

Frequency of Meals and Snacks

Not only is the *quantity* of food (calories) and its *quality* (ketogenic ratio and nutritional content) important, but also the *timing* of food intake can influence the success of the ketogenic diet.

As described in Chapter 1, an individual on a normal diet stores energy in the short term as glycogen and fat. During periods between eating or during starvation, the body first burns carbohydrate from food recently eaten, then burns carbohydrate that it has stored as glycogen, and finally begins to burn fat. Burning fat in the absence of carbohydrate results in ketosis.

Children on the ketogenic diet have virtually no carbohydrate in their diet, and they consume few calories, so they have virtually no stores of glycogen. Therefore, they depend on fat for their energy.

A child who is at her desirable weight has very little stored fat and therefore is dependent on the fats she eats at each meal. If too long a time passes between meals, the child may run out of fat to burn. Her

TABLE 5-1

The Content of Fats

	Grams	Protein	Fat	Carb	Kcal
Butter	100	0.67	81.33	0.00	735
Margarine, stick corn	100	0.00	76.00	0.00	684
Mayonnaise, Hellman's	100	1.43	80.00	0.70	729
Corn oil	100	0.00	97.14	0.00	874
Olive oil	100	0.00	96.43	0.00	868
Canola oil	100	0.00	90.00	0.00	810
Flaxseed oil	100	0.00	100.00	0.00	900
Peanut oil	100	0.00	96.43	0.00	868
MCT oil	100	0.00	92.67	0.00	834
Safflower oil	100	0.00	97.14	0.00	874

body will then burn some of its stored protein, but this will make her ketones decrease, and seizures may result.

WILLIAM WAS A 3-YEAR-OLD who was doing very well on the diet. His seizures decreased dramatically, but his parents noticed that he continued to have a few seizures early in the morning, before he woke up. William's ketones always measured very low in the morning, which the ketoteam interpreted as a sign that he needed to spread out his food intake. These early morning seizures disappeared after his dietitian calculated a late-night snack into William's diet.

Children usually have breakfast in the early morning and eat lunch around noon, but dinnertime is very variable. Some children are fed supper as early as 5:30 P.M. and then go to bed at 7:30–8:00 P.M. This means that they will not have eaten for 12 to 14 hours before their breakfast. This makes little difference to a child on a normal diet, who has plenty of energy reserves stored as glycogen and fat. But a child on the ketogenic diet may not have sufficient reserves to maintain ketosis overnight. If a child eats dinner later or has a snack at bedtime, the body is less likely to run out of ketones during the night. This may help to control early morning seizures.

Nutrasweet

Nutrasweet has been reported by some parents to induce seizures. If the parents suspect that Nutrasweet is causing their child's seizures, we ask that they test this by withholding it for a week or two and observing seizure frequency when the Nutrasweet is stopped. If seizure frequency increases when Nutrasweet is again reintroduced, it should be avoided. Avoiding Nutrasweet limits the flexibility of using readily available diet sodas, since most carbohydrate-free drinks are made with it. Parents can make drinks using saccharin instead if desired.

Changing the Diet's Ketogenic Ratio

Raising the diet's ratio [fat-to-(protein + carbohydrate)] increases the amount of fats consumed, with the goal of increasing ketosis and thereby resulting in better seizure control. If a child is continuing to have seizures, and if careful, thorough sleuthing has not revealed a cause, then raising the ketogenic ratio may be considered. We raise ratios in half-point increments, from 3:1 to 3.5:1, or from 4:1 to 4.5:1.

A 5:1 ketogenic ratio can occasionally be used for a few months, but it is so restrictive and so barely nutritionally adequate that we do not maintain it for more than a six-month period. We prefer the lowest ratio adequate to produce deep ketosis and seizure control.

Occasionally the ratio is decreased during the fine-tuning period if a child becomes anorexic and will not eat; if she remains too acidotic; if she is experiencing frequent illnesses; or if she is having persistent digestive difficulties on the diet. Most children start the diet on a 4:1 ratio. They are then adjusted down slowly after their first year on the diet.

Overweight children are an exception to this rule. We frequently start them on a diet in 3:1 ratio with restricted calories to facilitate weight loss. As they lose weight, they burn their own body fat, and this produces high ketones for them. As they approach their desirable weight, overweight children have less of their own body fat to burn, so we may need to increase the ratio to maintain the same high level of ketones.

MEDICATION LEVELS

The fine-tuning period usually involves adjusting medication levels as well as food and other non-food factors. Unless a child displays signs of overmedication, it is preferable to wait several weeks after initiation before tapering off medications. Only one medication should be tapered at a time, and diet changes should not be made at the same time as medication changes.

It is not uncommon for one or even a few breakthrough seizures to occur 24 to 72 hours after each decrease in medication dose. Parents should not reintroduce the medication or take any other action unless the seizures continue for more than a week. In this case reintroduction of the medication may be necessary. Benzodiazepines such as clonaze-

> **THE LIMITS OF FINE-TUNING** Not every child becomes seizure-free on the ketogenic diet. Not every child becomes medication-free. After working carefully with the ketoteam for several months, you will have to decide if there is enough improvement in your child's seizures, in his drug toxicity, in the child's life and your life to continue trying to make the diet even better. If you decide, together with the dietitian, that the child has received as much benefit from the diet as possible, then you will have to decide if that is good enough to continue. You can always go back to medication.

pam are addictive, and their withdrawal commonly produces seizures. For this reason, their reduction must be done very gradually to minimize withdrawal symptoms. A compounding pharmacy may be useful in preparing the increasingly dilute, sugar-free solutions needed for the weaning process.

Reducing anticonvulsant medications is a secondary but important goal of the ketogenic diet. Some children on the diet are able to stop taking all anticonvulsant medications and never have to go on them again. The situation varies for each individual.

Don't be in too much of a hurry to decrease or eliminate medications. Get the diet working first. When the family and child are on a stable routine, one medicine at a time can be gradually reduced and, if there is no recurrence of seizures, eliminated. If medication is reduced in this systematic, gradual fashion and the child does have a few seizures, it becomes easy to figure out the reason. The key to weaning children off their anticonvulsant medications during the fine-tuning period is to separate the effects of decreasing doses of medications from other factors in the diet. In other words, don't reduce medications at the same time as adjusting the food. Also, if a child has breakthrough seizures while the medicine is being reduced, don't assume that the seizures are a result of the tapering off. Look for all the possible factors and try to determine whether the reduction in medication is the cause.

BREAKTHROUGH SEIZURE ACTIVITY

As mentioned previously, the most common cause of breakthrough seizure activity in a child who is not ill and has been achieving good results on the ketogenic diet is that the child is getting the wrong amount of food or the wrong balance of food and liquid. Possible causes to look for include:

- The child is being given food that is not on the diet.
- The child is eating extra food in secret.
- The child has gained weight but not height—this indicates excess calories!
- The child has lost weight—calories are insufficient.
- Liquid is not being spaced out enough.
- Food is being improperly weighed or prepared.
- Information on food ingredients is incorrect.
- The diet has been miscalculated.
- The child is getting carbohydrates in toothpaste, sunscreen, or some other form.
- The child has come out of ketosis for some other reason.

The level of urinary ketosis may vary with the time of day. It is usually lower in the morning and higher later in the day. This natural variation in the level of ketones as measured in the urine does not necessarily indicate a problem if it is not accompanied by seizures.

If seizures do occur, parents, doctors, and dietitians should think about the elements of the diet and try to isolate possible causes for the breakthrough activity. The ketogenic diet decision tree described in Figure 5-1 can be used as a guide to this process.

The first thing to look for is whether the child has had an opportunity to eat something that is not on the diet. Food may have been given by someone or the child may have helped herself. One child was found to be sneaking sugared toothpaste in an upstairs bathroom. Another was slipping out of bed at night and raiding the refrigerator. Another girl had a seizure on Sunday, and her mother found to her dismay that she had been given a lollipop by a well-meaning grown-up at church.

Another possible cause of breakthrough activity on the diet is a calorie level that is set too high. If the body takes in more calories than are needed for maintenance, it will store those extra calories as fat. The body needs to burn all calories taken in to produce adequate ketosis and seizure control. Remember, the diet is simulating starvation, and you can't store calories when starving. As few as 100 calories too many per day can upset ketosis. In smaller infants, even 25 calories per day may be critical.

We will at times test the system in a child with low ketones by fasting the child for 24 hours. If the ketones rise after this fast, then we will decrease calories. Weight gain on the diet is an indication that calorie levels are set too high, with the exception of weight gain correlated to growth in height. At an excess of 100 calories per day, it takes an entire month before any weight gain is seen. Therefore, some caloric adjustments can be made based on low ketone levels.

Sometimes better control may be achieved by using a 4.5:1 ratio or even a 5:1 ratio for a period of time. The higher the diet ratio, the more restricted food options get, so the implications of raising the diet ratio should be seriously considered before it is prescribed.

The most common cause of breakthrough seizures in a child who is getting the proper food and liquid levels is illness or fever. An isolated seizure during illness requires no action on the part of the parents. Repeated breakthrough seizures can be the presenting sign of kidney stones, urinary tract infection, gastroenteritis, or other childhood infections. See Chapter 6 for greater detail on managing acute illness during the diet.

FIGURE 5-1

The Ketogenic Diet Decision Tree—for when a child with previous control begins having seizures

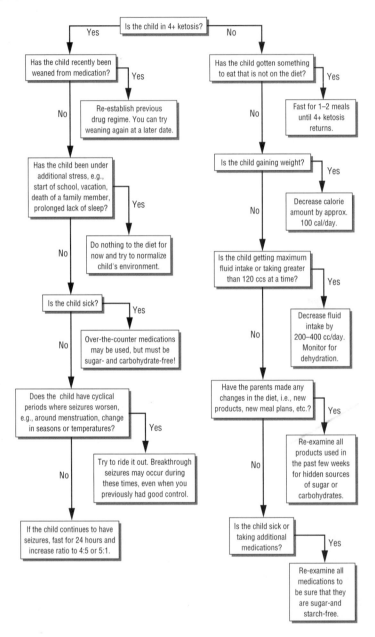

THERE MAY NOT BE A 100 PERCENT SOLUTION

In recent studies slightly more than half of children with difficult-to-control seizures find the ketogenic diet to be of sufficient benefit that they remain on the diet for more than one year. Not all of these are seizure-free! A reasonable aim for parents as their child starts on the ketogenic diet is to achieve as much seizure control as possible with as few medications as possible.

Improvements in behavior, mood, mental alertness, and a general sense of well-being are additional benefits that the diet often brings. If parents set a goal of total seizure control, they may be setting themselves up for disappointment. Total control may not be possible.

After trying the diet for the initial three-month period, and after working with the ketoteam to figure out if greater control can be achieved by adjusting food or medications, parents of children who have not responded to the diet or who have improved only moderately have to make a decision. These parents must weigh the benefits of the diet for their child against its burdens. Then they have to decide whether it is worthwhile for them to continue on the diet.

DON'T BE DAUNTED

If there are indications that a child is being helped by the diet but some problems remain, get into a fine-tuning mode. Be a sleuth. Parents, physicians, and dietitians must work together. Figure out the possible causes of the problems and root them out. Many children of intrepid, optimistic parents continue to improve over the entire course of the first year on the ketogenic diet.

CHAPTER SIX

MAKING IT WORK
AT HOME AND
ON THE ROAD

Be creative, but follow the rules exactly.
Follow the rules exactly, but be creative.

As long as you follow the rules exactly, but think creatively, you and your child can do just about anything you ever did before the diet started.

TIME-SAVERS

At first, most families find that the diet is very time-consuming to plan and prepare. But it gets faster and easier as you become accustomed to using the gram scale and planning meals in advance. We have estimated that in the first weeks, shopping and meal preparation may add an extra hour or two of commitment each day. But after this initial period, once you have gotten used to weighing food, parents say that preparing the diet may add a half-hour per day at most.

SHOPPING THE FIRST TIME TAKES FOREVER. Going up and down the aisles reading the fine print on each label searching for the words ending in "ose" or "ol" almost made me give up! But the second time was easier. Then I learned the brands I could use, and I only had to check to see that they hadn't changed the ingredients. —KM

Much time can be saved by preparing and storing meals or parts of meals in advance. You can refrigerate many foods for a few days or freeze them for a week or more. Following are some time-saving tips from parents who have experienced the diet:

- I cut up his favorite vegetables and keep them in plastic bags in the refrigerator for a few days. Then I can take them out and weigh a meal in no time.

- I usually make cream popsicles once a week. He has one after every dinner.

- We measure a day or two of meals at a time and put them in containers. That way we only have to do the weighing about every other day. Also, we can either serve the meals at home or take them with us if we are eating out.

- Whenever someone is celebrating a birthday at school, I know what to make for him—I send him in with a fruit-topped ketogenic cheesecake so he can have something good to eat, too.

- I put a cream shake in a container and freeze it so he can eat it later as ice cream or let it thaw back down to a shake.

- I always keep some tuna or chicken salad and bags of cut-up vegetables stored in the refrigerator in case I can't be there to fix dinner myself. He also takes these stored meals to school.

Be certain to label each meal or each part of a meal (Monday bkfst, Wednesday sup) before putting it in the refrigerator or the freezer so you remember what goes together.

GOING TO SCHOOL AND ON OTHER SHORT TRIPS

Anything the family did before they can still do on the diet—it will just take a little more planning. Every parent who has been through the diet has tips to offer:

- The key to making the diet "portable" is reusable storage containers.
- Cold food is easier to transport than hot food.
- It is easy to get food microwaved in a restaurant.
- It is usually easier to weigh and assemble a whole meal or several meals at home in advance than to weigh food on the road.

WITH BOTH OF US WORKING, and with all of the sports and church things for the other kids, finding time to make Brian's ketogenic meals was real hard. We finally found that if his mom and I worked together on Saturday morning, we could make all the meals for the week, label them, and put them in the freezer. Then at night we only had to make the family's supper—his was all ready to microwave.—KD

Eggnog is the traditional replacement meal, designed for all-purpose substitution in case of travel, sickness, or emergencies that make it difficult to prepare a meal. Eggnog is a complete meal-in-one (except for vitamin supplements), which is part of what makes it so convenient. Most children like the taste. Each sip is ketogenically balanced, so they don't have to drink all of it, or drink it all at once, to get its ketogenic effect.

Macadamia nuts, sometimes mixed with butter to achieve a higher ratio (they are naturally 3:1), can also be used as a meal-in-a-pinch or a travel meal or snack. A bag of chopped macadamia nuts drunk with a diet soda can be a very socially acceptable way for older children to eat around their friends, for instance on a field trip or sleepover.

Neither eggnog nor macadamia nuts should be used frequently in place of meals, because neither has enough protein or the nutritional value of regular meals with their meats, fruits, and vegetables. Both eggnog and macadamia nuts, however, can be extremely useful in a pinch.

> *WE CARRIED A SMALL COOLER with an ice pack in it everywhere. In the morning, we fixed the whole day's meal before going out. It got so that even if we weren't going anywhere we would set up all the meals for the day and stick them in Tupperware containers in the refrigerator. If we were going on a long trip, we would take about two days' worth of food with us in the cooler and bring our scale. Also, we always carried extra ingredients that we knew might be hard to buy, like olives. Everyone has a microwave, even on airplanes. We could give a fancy restaurant a couple of Tupperware containers and instructions for how long to cook things, and they would bring the food out on their own plate. Everybody was really cooperative. —RZ*

Following are some meal ideas for taking to school or on short outings. Each meal requires several reusable containers for storage.

- Tuna, chicken, or egg salad with mayonnaise
  Fresh vegetables (cucumber, carrot, cherry tomato, celery)
  Sugar-free Jell-O with whipped cream

- Celery or cucumber boats stuffed with tuna salad, cream cheese and butter, or peanut butter and butter
  Vanilla cream shake, whipped and frozen overnight

- Sandwich rolled in lettuce (chicken, cheese, turkey, or roast beef with mayonnaise)
  Water-packed canned peaches
  Chocolate milk (cream diluted with water and flavored with pure chocolate extract and saccharin)

- Cottage cheese with chopped fruit or vegetables and mayonnaise
  Cream shake, whipped and frozen overnight

- Fruit-topped "cheesecake," frozen overnight: a one-dish meal

FOODS FROZEN OVERNIGHT and taken out in the morning soften to a pudding-like consistency by lunchtime. Foods to be taken to school or on short outings can be wrapped in foil or carried in a thermal pouch or cooler for extra insulation to help stay either warm or cold. Whipped cream can be stored for a few hours and still keep its body.

When we went to Disneyland we just took a big cooler with three whole days of meals in labeled containers. Once we let him get a hot dog from the stand (which we then weighed) so he could feel like he was having a special treat. I wouldn't say it was easy doing all that planning, but for us it wasn't too difficult. —RZ

If you are going out to eat at a restaurant and you want your child to have a hot meal, call first to make sure the restaurant has a microwave that can be used for heating your food. If you are giving the child a cold meal, ask the restaurant to bring an extra plate, which will make the food look nice and add to the feeling of family togetherness. McDonald's will usually give a cup into which you can pour a sugar-free no-calorie soda. Bring your own can or bottle of soda, as diet drinks from the fountain may contain sorbitol.

DIET DON'TS

One mother kept her child out of school for a year and hired an in-home teacher because she did not want him to be tempted by seeing other children eat. Another family stopped going out entirely—no more McDonald's, no more Sunday dinners at grandma's—until the child himself finally begged them, explaining that he would enjoy the atmosphere and would not be too tempted by the food.

MANAGEMENT OF ACUTE ILLNESS DURING THE DIET

It may be difficult for a child who is sick to maintain ketosis. Sick children often do not feel like eating. Their activity level changes and they don't burn as many calories when they are ill. For these and other reasons many children on the diet experience a decrease in their urine ketone levels when sick. Seizure activity may increase at these times, or breakthrough seizures may occur even in children who have been well controlled on the diet. Parents can rest assured that ketosis will become reestablished as the illness resolves.

Helping your child to recover from an acute illness is more important than maintaining ketosis during times of illness! It may be necessary to break ketosis in order to treat an illness effectively. The most important thing is to get your child well again. The ketosis can be resumed once your child is well. The following are general guidelines for caring for a sick child on the ketogenic diet.

VOMITING OR DIARRHEA

- Give only sugar-free clear liquids. Do not worry about restricting fluids. Offer them frequently as tolerated.

- If vomiting lasts for more than 24 hours, use unflavored Pedialyte for up to 24 hours (but not longer) to maintain electrolytes.

- When vomiting stops you can introduce a 1/3 quantity eggnog meal. Each sip has the proper ketogenic ratio, and it is not necessary for your child to finish the eggnog if she does not want to. Increase as tolerated until the child is eating the full diet quantity. Then resume regular menus.

- If your child becomes dehydrated and IV fluids are required, make sure that they are sugar-free. If blood glucose is below 40, a single bolus of glucose (1 gram per kilogram of body weight) may be given.

- If your child is using MCT oil, discontinue until the illness is resolved. Substitute 1 gram canola or corn oil for each gram of MCT oil. The MCT oil can be resumed when your child is well.

Fever

- Give sugar-free fever-reducing medicine. Acetaminophen suppositories are an excellent fever reducer that won't interfere with the diet.

- Offer sugar-free liquids without restriction while your child has a fever.

- If an antibiotic is needed, make sure it is sugar-free and sorbitol-free. Speak with your pediatrician about using injectable antibiotics when possible, as a 7- to 10-day course of oral antibiotics may interfere with ketosis.

Too Much Ketosis

Sometimes a change in the diet or illness can cause children to get into too much ketosis. Some signs of too much ketosis are:

- rapid, panting (Kussmaul) breathing
- irritability
- increased heart rate
- facial flushing
- unusual fatigue or lethargy
- vomiting

If you suspect your child may be in too much ketosis, give him two tablespoons of orange juice. If the symptoms persist 20 minutes after giving the juice, give a second dose of two tablespoons orange juice. If the second dose of juice does not improve your child's condition, call your pediatrician and the supervising physician of your child's ketogenic diet immediately.

If you cannot reach the doctors, take your child to the emergency room. The emergency room doctors will check how acidotic your child has become. Intravenous fluids may be needed or even a dose of IV glucose to break up the excessive ketosis. In the meantime, ask the emergency room to continue trying to contact your ketoteam.

Sugar-Free Medication

Work with your pediatrician and local pharmacist to obtain any necessary medications in sugar-free and carbohydrate-free form. A list of medications is provided in Appendix A. If a medication you need is not commercially available in carbohydrate-free form, try contacting a compounding pharmacy such as New Jersey's Ridge Pharmacy (1-800-RIDGE RX) for custom-made medications.

BABYSITTERS AND OTHER PARENT-LESS MEALS

In most households, the person who usually prepares the meals is occasionally unavailable—working late, sick, at a party, or otherwise engaged. Not to worry! With a little planning, someone else can easily put a meal together from your prepared ingredients.

Many parents store measured ingredients or prepared food a couple of days ahead of time in the refrigerator even when they are planning to be present to prepare each meal. The habit of preparing meals in advance both saves time on a routine basis and makes it easier to cope with special situations. Just like with non-ketogenic meals, it rarely hurts to have something ready in the freezer.

Some items can be measured and stored or frozen up to a week in advance:

Popsicles	Beef
Cream shakes	Chicken
Cheesecake	Eggnog
Ice cream	Cut-up fresh vegetables
Sugar-free Jell-O	

Note that foods such as ice cream must be calculated and carefully labeled to go with a particular meal that you plan to make. This is because different meal plans use varying amounts of cream and ingredients such as fruit or oil may need to be frozen into the ice cream, depending on what else is being served for supper. Other foods can be prepared, weighed, and stored in the refrigerator one or two days in advance:

Cooked meat or chicken portions	D-Zerta gelatin
Tuna, egg, or chicken salads	Vegetables
Cream portions for whipping	Fresh fruit
Tomato sauce	Sliced or grated cheese

If a parent sets out measured ingredients and instructions, a sibling or babysitter can easily carry out final assembly of the meal. Make these meals simple: try to think of meals that can be put in one microwave dish and cooked or reheated (stew, squash/cheese/butter casserole) or meals that do not need cooking at all (tuna salad).

LONG TRIPS

Yes, the family can take vacations. Longer trips by necessity involve more planning than shorter ones. Many families who take long vacations choose to stay in places where they can cook, such as friends' condominiums or motels with kitchenettes, rather than in hotels. They sometimes take eggnog for the road instead of a solid meal. They take their scale and call ahead to make sure that places where they will be staying have heavy cream and a microwave available. With the scale, they can order grilled chicken, steamed vegetables, and mayonnaise and create a quick meal right at the restaurant.

Families take coolers full of prepared ingredients for the first couple of days of a trip, and perhaps staples such as artificial sweetener and mayonnaise. If they are staying in a hotel with no kitchen, they might take a camping stove to cook on. They take a lot of storage containers.

They take their calcium and multivitamin supplements, too, of course, because they never forget those.

Apart from the nuisance of planning, the diet should be no obstacle to family fun. There is no reason why a child should not live a rich, full, and healthy life while on the ketogenic diet.

HE SKIED THIS YEAR FOR THE FIRST TIME in ages. He skied like you wouldn't believe. He's swimming, he's playing ball. He's definitely had a happier life on the diet. —CC

B E CREATIVE

Being creative can mean compensating for a small quantity of cucumbers and carrots by slicing them in tall, thin strips and fanning them out to cover more plate space. It can mean dressing up the cream as a toasted almond ice cream, whipped into a mound, flavored with almond extract and sweetener, and sprinkled with a crushed almond. Let the child sprinkle on the nuts for fun.

There are lots of calorie-free ways to keep the food lively. Play with variables that add interest, not calories:

- shapes
- natural food colors or food coloring
- herbs and spices (just a tiny pinch because these have carbohydrates)
- pure flavoring extracts
- pretending

Of course, many children do not care about variety and whimsy in their food. Some children are comforted by regularity. We have seen many families cook the same six meals over and over for two years, and the child was perfectly content.

WE FREEZE HIS DIET DECAFFEINATED POP in miniature ice cube trays. They make refreshing little treats. He has a small amount as a goodie before bedtime. We give it to him in a wine glass to make it fancy and special. We also make popsicles out of his pop. If it's clear pop, we let him mix in food coloring drops, so he is not only involved but also learning. This adds lots of laughs when his teeth and lips turn green or blue or purple.—EH

Peaches can be swapped for strawberries, broccoli for spinach. Combine fruits or vegetables for variety—peaches with a couple of raspberries on top, or asparagus with carrots. Switching the foods around helps add variety to the meals. If a child wants variety, there's plenty of room for creativity within the diet.

> *HE HAS HIS SPECIAL "PIZZA." It's just cheese and ground beef melted on a thin slice of tomato, cut into triangles the shape of pizza slices. But he loves it. It's pizza to him! —EH*

FOLLOW THE RULES EXACTLY

If the rules are followed exactly, the family will know the child was given the best possible chance to obtain the maximum benefits of the diet. Being very strict helps the ketoteam know where a child stands with the diet. The effect of the ketogenic diet is directly related to the food that is eaten and the liquid that is drunk. This may seem obvious, but it is the factor that makes the diet work.

Especially when using commercial products, knowing the precise content of the food is essential. Buy the exact brand specified by the dietitian. The same product, such as bologna, made by different manufacturers may have very different proportions of protein, fat, and carbohydrates. The dietitian will have based diet calculations on the proportions of a given brand, so if a new brand is used, the calculations may have to be changed.

> *ABOUT A WEEK AFTER HE STARTED THE DIET, my son was doing great. Then we went to the store and bought some commercial turkey loaf. The meal plan called for turkey, so we thought turkey loaf would be just as good. Well, I don't know what was in it, but my son had a very bad day the next day. That's when we discovered that when the meal plan says turkey, it means plain, fresh turkey, not turkey loaf. You have to follow instructions to the letter. —FD*

If a different brand needs to be introduced, the parents or dietitian must research the product carefully, even if it means calling the manufacturer to find out. Make sure that the new brand is properly calculated into the meal plans.

It WOULD NEVER HAVE OCCURRED TO US to eat something that wasn't allowed on the diet. Even when we were allowed to, when the diet was ending, we had a hard time imagining eating food that hadn't been allowed before. —CC

Even when a commercial product is known and used regularly, formulations and commercial recipes can change. If breakthrough seizures develop, this should be one source of suspicion. At the risk of repeating ourselves, ingredients of commercially prepared foods, which are beyond your power to control, have to be watched very carefully. Be cautious in reading labels as well. By law, products that contain less than 1 gram of an ingredient per serving may be listed as zero, so a product that you thought had no carbohydrates may actually have up to 0.9 grams. If used on a regular basis, this can add up to a lot of excess carbohydrates. With basic ingredients such as fresh meat, fruit, and vegetables, this is not much of a problem, although the exact content of even fresh produce does vary slightly from one source to another.

If your child is having problems with the diet, always consider the food—both its quantity and its content—as the most likely culprit.

Are there commercial products in the diet? Has the source of cream or bacon changed? Is the cream still 36 percent to 40 percent fat? Different children have different amounts of tolerance for variations in food content. It is the little things that often spell the difference between success and failure of the diet. If your child is doing well on the diet, obviously you shouldn't worry. You should simply continue to be careful.

THERE WAS ONE TIME we wanted to try a new brand of sausage. We read the label very carefully and checked it with Mrs. Kelly and everything. But shortly after we started including it in her diet, our daughter began feeling shaky, what she described as "wobbly" inside. Dr. Freeman said it sounded like she might be trying to break through with seizures. We're pretty sure it was because of that sausage; either the label was wrong or it referred to raw quantities and we were using cooked, or something. We went back to the old brand, and then she was fine. —MH

GET THE WHOLE FAMILY INVOLVED

You and your child are making a tremendous effort to stick to the diet in pursuit of a tremendous goal, and you need everyone's cooperation and encouragement. You can weigh the food in advance, but if you are not there at dinnertime, someone else—an older sister or brother, a sitter, a grandmother—can put it in the microwave and serve the meal.

A child on the diet and all the child's sisters and brothers, relatives, friends, and teachers should understand that even tiny amounts of cheating can spoil the overall effect of the diet, and that their friendship, support, and encouragement are crucial to its success.

THE INTERNET

The Internet is an increasingly common source of information and support for parents of children with health problems, including epilepsy. The feedback we receive from parents who use the Internet to obtain information about the ketogenic diet indicates that this information is of greatly varying quality.

- Some of the information is excellent and very valuable.
- Some of the information is incorrect and/or misleading.
- Some of the information shows the bias of an enthusiastic parent.
- Some of the information shows the bias of a disgruntled parent.

If you use or intend to use the Internet as a source of information on the ketogenic diet, be aware of the varying quality of information you may be receiving. Keep in mind the source of the information. The challenge is to separate the useful information on the ketogenic diet from that which is incorrect.

EVERYTHING WENT REALLY WELL FOR US. We were really careful, read every label, never gave her anything that wasn't allowed. We followed the rules to the Nth degree. And she never had any more seizures. —MH

GOING OFF
THE DIET

Children who get good benefit from the ketogenic diet traditionally remain on the 4:1 ketogenic ratio for two years or until they have been seizure-free without medication for one full year. Then they switch to a 3:1 diet ratio for six months. If they remain seizure-free, this is followed by a 2:1 ratio for six months, after which they are weaned off the diet and can eat any foods they want.

The above schedule is somewhat arbitrary. There are as yet no studies of the best ways of discontinuing the diet. The two-year time figure is the result of tradition rather than science, although studies of diet discontinuation are in progress.

Approximately 29 percent of children who start on the diet discontinue it within six months of initiation because the diet is ineffective, too difficult, or for other reasons. If the family and ketoteam determine that the ketogenic diet is not the best therapy for a child, the discontinuation increments can be taken more rapidly, normally over a period of weeks.

If a serious medical problem or other special situation arises, the ketoteam will determine the most effective way of discontinuing the diet. In all cases, discontinuation of the diet should be carried out under the guidance of a trained ketoteam.

The traditional regimen for easing off the diet over the course of a year may be more cautious than is absolutely necessary, but we believe it is better to err on the side of caution. There has been concern (although without much evidence) that withdrawing too abruptly from the diet could bring back seizures, and possibly even status epilepticus, wiping out all those months of discipline.

The length of time a child has to stay on the 4:1 ratio is sometimes extended by a year or two if a child has not stuck to the regimen strictly or if there is some other reason to think more time on the diet will help the child. For some children whose seizures have not been completely controlled, it is possible to continue the diet beyond two years to maintain the degree of control that has been achieved. **Clearly, the diet does not have to be discontinued after two years.** Continuing the diet in this case is an alternative to the increased medications that will probably be needed when the diet is stopped.

If a child who has been well controlled on the diet begins to have seizures again once it has ended (this is very rare), it is possible to restart the diet.

There has been no research indicating a strong chemical or metabolic reason for stopping the diet after two successful years rather than staying on it longer; it is just good to get back to a normal life.

The question of when to discontinue the diet is particularly urgent for the many children whose seizures are 50 percent to 90 percent or more improved, but who are not made seizure-free by the diet. Will their seizures recur after discontinuation? Will medications have to be reinstituted? These are questions that remain to be studied.

BEN HAS BEEN ON THE DIET FOR NINE YEARS NOW. He is severely retarded and fed by gastrostomy. His cholesterol is 116. He has had no seizures in more than eight years. His mother says "Taper the diet? Why would we do that? The diet is no trouble for us and makes no difference to Ben."

The long-term consequences of remaining on the ketogenic diet for many years have not yet been studied. Some handicapped children have been maintained on the diet for many years without obvious ill effects. Studies have shown that lipids and triglycerides are elevated during the diet to levels that would normally be considered to increase the threat of stroke or heart disease after a lifetime of exposure. The potential threat of stroke or heart disease after a limited exposure of two or even ten years of a high-fat diet has not been studied. Any health threat would have to be evaluated in relation to alternative health risks posed by uncontrolled epilepsy, such as increased seizures or increased long-term intake of anticonvulsant medications.

I HAD NOT SEEN OR HEARD FROM TYLER in many years when his family called to ask if they could increase his calories. We asked them to come to the clinic. Tyler was now a late teenager, with cerebral palsy and moderate retardation. He had been on the diet for 15 years. He had grown and was doing well but still had one or two seizures per year. He was on no medications, and the family did not want to use any. "He's doing just fine on the diet," they said. "We just want him to gain a bit of weight." —JMF

The decision to come off the diet is for the most part left to the parents. Some, especially those for whom the diet's benefits are incremental, wonder early on whether the diet is worth the trouble. They want to know what the difference would be if their child was on a normal diet. For these parents, we sometimes suggest substituting whole milk for the heavy cream over a two-week trial period. This is roughly equivalent to switching to a 3:1 ketogenic ratio and is easy to undo because it does not disrupt the diet's ritual. (Going off the diet entirely for two weeks, on the other hand, may permanently alter the child's or family's willingness to comply with the diet's rigors.)

If there is no change in seizure activity during the following week or two, then we suggest substituting skim milk for the whole milk. This is approximately the equivalent of going to a 2:1 ketogenic ratio. If seizure activity does not change over the next week or so, then the family often chooses to discontinue the diet entirely. While we have not assessed this plan in a rigorous fashion, it may provide a useful alternative to recalculating meal plans in order to let a borderline family test discontinuation of the diet.

Deborah returned for her three-month follow-up visit.
While the diet had substantially reduced her seizures and had allowed her to stop one of her medications, both Deborah and her mother were finding it very difficult. They wanted to discontinue the diet. We suggested substituting whole milk for the cream for a two-week trial. After only one week Deborah's mother called to ask if she could switch back to cream, as Deborah's seizures had grown much worse since switching to milk. —JMF

Some children who have responded exceptionally well to the diet also start to come off it before the two-year mark is reached. This decision is often suggested by the parents and agreed to in consultation with the physicians.

Toward the end we started letting him smell things. The other kids would give him a sniff of what they were eating and he would say, "I can have that when I'm off the diet, right?" —CC

She was a junior bridesmaid at a wedding the day she went off the diet. That was when she was twelve. We had checked with Mrs. Kelly and agreed to let her eat cake at the reception. All of us were very apprehensive. There had been a lot of anxiety each time we cut the ratio, but she kept doing well, so sweets were the last test. Nobody else at the reception really knew what we were going through—it was a private thing among us and our very close friends. When she ate the cake and had no problems, it was thrilling for us. After that we were probably cautious for another week or two. Now she won't look at whipped cream, but she eats just like a typical teenager—pizza and candy and all the typical teenage food. —MH

We had been down to a 1:1 ratio for a few months when one day [the doctor] said, "Why don't you take him out for an ice cream sundae— you're off the diet!" Well, I couldn't quite do that but we did take him for a steak and potato dinner. Then about an hour later I got him a little dish of mint chocolate chip ice cream. It was very dramatic for me to see him eat a real meal. And for him, too—his little eyes were watering. It was a tear-jerking experience. We had finally made it! He used to be an extremely picky eater but now he just really enjoys eating. —JS

AFTER HE HAD DONE PERFECTLY *for a year and a half on the 4:1 diet, we had done six months on the 3:1, and then a couple of months on the 2:1, when his sixth birthday was coming up. We asked him what he wanted, and he said pizza. Well, you're nervous as can be, but he was doing so well that we decided to stop the diet on his birthday, before the full six months of the 2:1 were up. We invited all the neighborhood kids in, and I put candles in the pizza. After he took the first bite, he looked up at me and said, "Dad, this is the best birthday present I've ever had." —RZ*

ANXIETY AND RELIEF

It is natural for a parent to feel anxious when a child is going off the diet. After all that time spent planning and measuring food to an accuracy of a gram, it's hard to kick the habit! All we can tell nervous parents is that ending the diet is to their child's advantage once the child is seizure-free for two years. The ketogenic diet therapy's goal is to treat a problem—seizures. Once the problem is gone, the therapy should also end.

A child can start going off the diet once the full benefits of the diet have been realized. Exactly when this invisible finish line has been crossed will vary for each child. But by the time a child has been on the diet rigidly for two years and is seizure-free, its long-term benefits will most likely have already been gained. If the EEG has returned to normal, for instance, it is likely to stay normal. Even if the EEG is still abnormal, it may be possible for the child who has been seizure-free for two years to go off the diet gradually without the return of seizures. The child is likely to remain seizure-free when normal eating is resumed if there have been no seizures with no medication during the diet.

AFTER WE HAD BEEN ON THE 2:1 DIET *for about six weeks I asked what was next, and Mrs. Kelly said I could give him some popcorn with lots of butter. I was so nervous I was shaking when I gave it to him. He felt the same way. "Are you sure she said I could have popcorn?" he asked me.*

I almost didn't know how to gradually withdraw the diet. When it came time to go off it, the thought of giving him a glass of low-fat milk instead of cream made me crazy with nerves. —CC

GOING OFF THE DIET WAS VERY LIBERATING. *At last we could go places without planning and thinking about every meal. We could spend a day at the mall. She could go to parties and eat what the other kids were having. It was great.* —MH

Lower ketogenic ratios are increasingly similar to regular meals. A 2:1 ratio will seem almost like a normal diet compared with the 4:1. There will be room for a lot more meat and vegetables and even the possibility of some carbohydrates.

Once a child has been weaned down to a 2:1 ratio and has been on that ratio for a few months, we recommend that formerly forbidden foods be gradually introduced into the diet. We encourage parents to start with somewhat fatty foods, such as buttery popcorn, greasy french fries, and hamburgers. Sometimes we go to a 1:1 ratio for a few months, which can be useful as a tapering method even though at this ratio the child is no longer in ketosis. In general, though, when the gradually introduced foods have reached a point where the child is no longer in ketosis, you're home free!

FOR ME THE DIET REALLY WASN'T ALL THAT HARD. *There wasn't a single day when I resented having to weigh the meals. For me it was a very pleasant experience. It was just a miracle.* —JS

SECTION III

CALCULATIONS

CHAPTER EIGHT

CALCULATING THE KETOGENIC DIET

The initial ketogenic diet prescription is three parts science and one part art. It requires a full nutritional assessment and an understanding of the child's medical condition, combined with prioritization, empathy, and intuition. In each case, a child's individual needs must be taken into account.

ESTIMATING CALORIC NEEDS

In calculating the caloric requirements of an individual child, one must consider not only the child's current and desirable weight but also her activity level. The estimated calorie needs for infants and children as published in *The Nutrition Manual for At-risk Infants and Toddlers* is shown in Table 8-1. These recommendations are for average children with average activity levels.

As indicated in Table 8-1, the basal metabolic rate for a child one to two years of age is 40 kcal/kg. Then 17 kcal/kg are added for specific

TABLE 8-1

Estimating Calorie Needs for Infants and Children

Age (yr)	BMR (kcal/kg)	SDA+EXC (kcal/kg)	Activity (kcal/kg)	Growth (kcal/kg)	Total (kcal/kg)
0–0.5	55	20	17	20	112
0.5–1	55	17	20	13	105
1–2	40	17	22	11	90
3–4	40	14	21	10	85

BMR = Basal metabolic rate, which is similar to REE + < 10%; it is this component of energy expenditure that is increased during fever or other stress

SDA = Specific dynamic action or energy required for digestion and absorption

EXC = Energy lost through excretion

Note: Energy levels vary greatly, depending on activity levels, stage of growth phase, and individual constitution. It is usually recommended that ideal weight for length or height ("expected" weight for length or height or 50th percentile weight for length or height) be used to calculate caloric needs. However, if muscle mass is lower or higher than normal, estimated "lean body weight" may be used.

Reference: Lowrey, *Growth and Development in Children,* 6th ed. Chicago: Year Book, 1973.

Source: The Nutrition Manual for At-risk Infants and Toddlers. Precept Press, 1992, p. 231.

dynamic action, 22 kcal for activity, and 11 kcal for growth. The caloric requirement for an average one-year-old child is therefore 90 kcal/kg (40 + 17 + 22 + 11 = 90).

The ketogenic diet is generally based on 75 percent of Recommended Daily Allowance (RDA) of calories for a child's desirable weight and height, but it can be modified to allow for such factors as the child's activity level, natural rate of metabolism, and local climate.

The goal of the diet is to provide optimal seizure control and maintain adequate nutrition for the child. When we make our initial estimates of the child's dietary needs, we begin by assessing his age, weight, height, health, and activity status. The ketogenic diet appears to work best when the child is neither too fat nor too lean and when she is close to her "desirable body weight." This is defined as the 50th percentile of weight for height. Overweight children need to lose weight. Underweight children need to gain to their ideal weight. At the desirable weight there is sufficient fat reserve for the child to burn between meals. If there is too much body fat, the child will rarely become sufficiently ketotic to control seizures. We therefore use desirable weight for height as an input in estimating a child's caloric needs.

That is just the start, however, since the child's activity level is also an important determinant of her caloric needs. A very active child needs more calories than a less active one. Profoundly handicapped children, who sometimes are very inactive, usually require fewer calories per kilogram than an average child. In such handicapped children, a diet calculated for their desirable body weight will cause them to gain weight and will not provide sufficient ketosis.

Providing approximately 75 percent of the calories normally recommended for the child's age and desirable weight should be enough to allow most children to grow normally and remain close to their desirable weight for their age and height. They should neither gain nor lose disproportionate weight for at least the first year on the diet.

Protein

RDAs are calculated for average children of a given height and weight and an average activity level. The ketogenic diet, however, is rarely used for average children. Protein is set at 1 gram per kilogram of body weight except in small, rapidly growing children, in whom we strive for 1.5 grams per kilogram. In adolescents it may be difficult to achieve the proper fat:carbohydrate ratio if 1 gram/kilo of protein is given, and we may use as little as 0.75 grams of protein per kilogram. We use RDA and World Health Standards as guidelines (Table 8-2). Growth is closely monitored and is used as a guide of adequate nutrition.

The most important factor in the successful and safe initiation of the diet is close contact between the family and the ketogenic diet team during the early weeks.

Given that a detailed nutritional assessment and lab work are essential to the initial diet prescription, there are four main areas to which the

TABLE 8-2

Protein Allowances

Age	RDA for Protein (g/kg)	WHO Mean Protein Allowance (g/kg)
0–6 months	2.2	1.38
6–12 months	1.6	1.21
1–3 years	1.2	0.97
4–6 years	1.1	0.84
7–10 years	1.0	0.80
Males 11–14 yrs	1.0	0.79
Males 15–18 yrs	0.9	0.69
Females 11–14 yrs	1.0	0.76
Females 15–18 yrs	0.8	0.64
Adults	0.8	—

Source: *Recommended Dietary Allowances,* 10th edition. Washington, DC: National Academy Press, 1989.

physician's and dietitian's judgment must be applied in determining the input values for the ketogenic diet calculation:

- desirable weight vs. actual weight
- calories per kilogram
- ketogenic ratio (fat:protein + carbohydrate)
- fluid allotment

Although the diet traditionally approximated 75 percent of RDAs, individualized caloric values based on current/desirable weight and activity levels will provide better nutrition.

The initial ketogenic ratio is usually 4:1 unless a child is very young or very overweight, or has a very fragile medical condition. In the case of a very overweight child, the 3:1 diet will be based on a desirable weight lower than the current weight, and this should lead to some weight loss.

In the case of the child who is substantially underweight, you may want to base the child's calories/kilogram on the *current* weight and then

CHILDREN SHOULD BE WEIGHED every week and the weights written down by the parents or recorded on a growth chart. Weights should be taken at the same time of day, prior to a meal, and without clothes. If there is excess weight gain, the child is receiving too many calories. If there is excess weight loss, the calories may need to be increased. Over the longer term children should gain weight in proportion to their growth in height. Children should be measured every three months in their physician's office, their height and weight plotted on a growth chart, and calories should be adjusted to keep weight proportional to growth.

slowly increase the calories by small increments. A child with feeding problems or recurrent aspiration may benefit from a feeding tube or gastrostomy before starting the diet.

Fluid Allotment

Although fluid restriction has not been well studied and its importance to the diet is not entirely clear, anecdotal evidence indicates that fluid intake levels may affect seizure control in children on the ketogenic diet. Fluid allotments are set at about 80 percent of maintenance for healthy, active children:

BODY WEIGHT	FLUID ALLOTMENT
1–10 kg	80 ml/kg
10–20 kg	800 ml + 40 ml/kg
>20 kg	1200 ml + 20 ml/kg

Fluid allocation should be individualized and increased with an increase in activity or a hot climate. Fluids are not restricted during illness and are increased to 100 ml/kg for fragile children and infants under one year of age.

Urine specific gravity should be 1.010–1.020 and may be used as a guide to adequate hydration.

THE CASE OF JAMES

The following case illustrates the thought process of a dietitian in evaluating an individual coming in for ketogenic diet initiation:

James is a 4-year-7-month-old male with history of infantile spasms (myoclonic seizures) and developmental delay. Seizure onset was at 12 months of age. Seizure frequency is 100–150 jerks/day.

CURRENT MEDICATIONS: Topamax 75 mg BID, Depakote 375 mg TID, Tranxene 0.9 mg daily. Supplements: Bugs Bunny multivitamin/mineral.

LABS: No current labs available.

FEEDING ABILITY: No impairment—James feeds himself—no problems with chewing, swallowing, etc. No history of pneumonia or aspiration.

James's mother reports his appetite to be poor and states that he is a "picky eater." James normally eats a great deal of starches (pasta, bread, etc.) as well as vegetables. He does not like meat very much. He eats three meals and two snacks daily. Food preferences recorded. Activity is low to normal—James participates in phys ed once a week and recess at school. His bowel movements are normal for the most part. No known food allergies or intolerances.

THREE-DAY FOOD RECALL: Average intake 1,290 kcal, 42 gm vitamin/mineral consumption adequate with the exception of calcium.

WT: 18.4 kg, Ht 111.8 cm (40.5 lbs, 44 inches)

WT FOR AGE: 50–75%

HT FOR AGE: 75–90%

WT FOR HT: 25–50%

Ideal Body Wt at 19.4 kg (wt for ht at 50%)
James is 95% of Ideal Body Weight

James's growth pattern has been relatively normal—both height and weight were proportional following the 75 percent to 90 percent curve until six months ago. His mother said that James has been the same weight for six months now, despite an increase in height. She attributes his lack of weight gain to a decreased appetite since the addition of Topamax.

PHYSICAL ASSESSMENT: No physical signs of deficiencies. James appears to be well nourished, although quite lean.

Assessment

James does not appear to be at nutritional risk at this point. Despite not gaining weight for six months, he is still 95 percent of his ideal weight, and weight has crossed only one percentile. He looks healthy, is consuming what is recommended for age for protein, macro- and micronutrients (with the exception of calcium intake of only 700 mg). Caloric intake is obviously too low as seen by the lack of weight gain and the fact that the child is under his ideal body weight. It is reasonable to start him at his current caloric intake at a 4:1 ratio. We do not want him to lose weight, and the high ratio will allow us to provide the fat needed for ketosis via the diet.

Initial Diet

1,300 kcal, 4:1 ratio, 1,200 cc total fluid daily. To be given in three equal meals and a snack of 150 kcal before bedtime.

KCAL: 1,300 (70.7 kcal/kg ideal body weight)

TOTAL PROTEIN: 24.5 gm (1.3 gm/kg ideal body weight)

TOTAL CARBOHYDRATE: 8 gm

TOTAL FAT: 130 gm

TOTAL FLUID: 1,200 cc (80 percent of estimated maintenance needs)

Goals

1. Seizure control.
2. Attaining ideal weight within three-month period. Increasing kcal in small increments (5 percent to 10 percent of kcal every

2 to 4 weeks) while weaning some medication should be sufficient to attain this goal provided that seizures are well controlled. James will probably not only have improvement of
appetite, but hopefully of activity as well if his seizures can be
controlled.

3. Maintaining optimal nutritional status (maintaining growth and
   overall nutritional status long term).

Plan

1. Implement diet, educate parents.
2. Attain biochemical indices to check nutritional status (visceral
   protein status, anemias, electrolytes, hydration, renal function,
   etc.).
3. Discuss Topamax wean with physicians. Weaning this medication aggressively could help with the child's side effects
   (anorexia).
4. Order multivitamin/mineral supplement that meets patient's
   recommended micronutrient needs 100 percent.
5. Continue to track height, weight, seizure control, etc. via phone.
6. See James at three-month follow-up visit.

Once judgments are made about ideal weight, ketogenic ratio, and
liquid allotment, the ketogenic diet can be calculated. Although the
computer software makes calculating the menus much faster and easier,
it is useful to understand the steps of the calculation so that it can be
modified if necessary to meet a child's individual needs.

GENERAL RULES FOR THE INITIAL KETOGENIC DIET CALCULATION

1. Decide on an optimal level of calories. This should be done
   using a thorough medical and nutritional history and the dietitian and physician's professional judgment. Variables such as the

child's activity level, frame size, medical condition, recent weight gain or loss, etc. must be taken into account.

2. Set the desired ketogenic ratio. Most children are started on a 4:1 ketogenic ratio. Very overweight or medically compromised children may be started on a 3:1 or 3.5:1 ratio of fat:protein + carbohydrates. Children under two years of age and adolescents are usually started on a 3:1 ratio.

3. Liquid levels should be set at about 80 percent of maintenance for healthy, active children as described on p. 123. Liquids are increased for fragile children and infants under one year of age. Urine specific gravity may be used as a guide to adequate hydration.

4. Always strive to attain RDAs for protein (1.1–1.5 gm/kg), and never allow protein to fall below World Health Organization standards.

5. The ketogenic diet must be supplemented daily with calcium and a sugar-free, lactose-free multivitamin with minerals. The diet is not nutritionally sufficient without supplementation.

Since this book is written for parents and medical professionals, and since we believe that the diet works best with informed parents as part of the team, we believe it is important to know as much about the diet as possible. **BUT: The ketogenic diet should never be attempted without careful medical and nutritional supervision.**

ROSEANNE WAS 5 YEARS OLD when she was admitted to the intensive care unit with pneumonia, dehydration , and a very low pulse rate. There were major concerns about whether she would survive the night. She appeared wasted, cachectic, and looked as though she had been starved by her parents. The nurse called the child abuse team. The parents arrived a few minutes later, having followed the ambulance from the referring hospital. They seemed very nice and very concerned. They said that Roseanne had suffered from lack of oxygen at birth and was quite developmentally delayed. She still could not sit by herself or communicate. Roseanne had seizures beginning at six months old and had been treated with many medications, but without much success. The parents had come to the con-clusion that not only were the medications not helping, but their side effects were part of the reason for Roseanne's lack of progress. "All those doctors were doing was experimenting on our daughter," they said.

"We saw this program on TV about some sort of diet for the epilepsy that would get you off the medications. We called Hopkins, but they couldn't do the diet on her for three months, and we couldn't wait that long. So we did it ourselves. It wasn't so hard, and the seizures were better, until the last month when she just didn't seem to want to eat. Then the past few days she started throwing up and breathing real funny. I guess now you'll have to take her!"

Roseanne had pneumonia, but was also severely acidotic, malnourished, and dehydrated. With intensive care over the following week she gradually came around and was able to be discharged home, not on the diet. Until she had built up her reserves and had become better nourished, we felt that the diet posed too much of a risk. This was not a case of child abuse, but rather one of frustration with the medical profession and an impatience with the processes involved. It almost resulted in the child's death.

HOW A DIETITIAN CALCULATES THE DIET: AN EXAMPLE

1. AGE AND WEIGHT. Fill out the following information:

Age _____

Desirable weight in kilograms _____

Mary has been prescribed a 4:1 ketogenic diet. She is four years old and currently weighs 15 kilograms (33 pounds). Her dietitian has determined that this weight is appropriate for Mary.

2. CALORIES PER KILOGRAM. After a full medical and nutritional assessment, a dietitian will assign a calorie per kilogram level for diet initiation.

The dietitian has set Mary's prescription at 68 kcal/kg. Note that this figure involves a dietitian's judgment; it is slightly higher than

75 percent of caloric needs if estimated from Table 8.1 (85 kcal/kg $\times$ 0.75 = 64 kcal/kg).

3. TOTAL CALORIES. Determine the total number of calories in the diet by multiplying the child's weight by the number of calories set per kilogram.

Mary, age four and weighing 15 kilograms, needs a total of 68 $\times$ 15 or 1,020 calories per day.

4. DIETARY UNIT COMPOSITION. Dietary units are the building blocks of the ketogenic diet. A 4:1 diet has dietary units made up of 4 grams of fat to each 1 gram of protein + carbohydrate. Because fat has 9 calories per gram (9 $\times$ 4 = 36), and protein and carbohydrate each have 4 calories per gram (4 $\times$ 1 = 4), a dietary unit at a 4:1 diet ratio has 36 + 4 = 40 calories. The caloric value and breakdown of dietary units vary with the ketogenic ratio:

RATIO	FAT CALORIES	CARBOHYDRATE PLUS PROTEIN CALORIES	CALORIES PER DIETARY UNIT
2:1	2 g $\times$ 9 kcal/g = 18	1 g $\times$ 4 kcal/g = 4	18 + 4 = 22
3:1	3 g $\times$ 9 kcal/g = 27	1 g $\times$ 4 kcal/g = 4	27 + 4 = 31
4:1	4 g $\times$ 9 kcal/g = 36	1 g $\times$ 4 kcal/g = 4	36 + 4 = 40
5:1	5 g $\times$ 9 kcal/g = 45	1 g $\times$ 4 kcal/g = 4	45 + 4 = 49

Mary's dietary units will be made up of 40 calories each because she is on a 4:1 ratio.

5. DIETARY UNIT QUANTITY. Divide the total calories allotted (Step 3) by the number of calories in each dietary unit (Step 4) to determine the number of dietary units to be allowed daily.

Each of Mary's dietary units on a 4:1 ratio contains 40 calories, and she is allowed a total of 1,020 kcal/day, so she gets 1,020/40 = 25.5 dietary units per day.

6. FAT ALLOWANCE. Multiply the number of dietary units by the units of fat in the prescribed ketogenic ratio to determine the grams of fat permitted daily.

On her 4:1 diet, with 25.5 dietary units/day, Mary will have 25.5 × 4 or 102 grams of fat per day.

7. PROTEIN + CARBOHYDRATE ALLOWANCE. Multiply the number of dietary units by the number of units of protein + carbohydrate in the prescribed ketogenic ratio, usually one, to determine the combined daily protein + carbohydrate allotment.

On her 4:1 diet, Mary will have 25.5 × 1 or 25.5 grams of protein + carbohydrate per day.

8. PROTEIN ALLOWANCE. The dietitian will determine optimal protein levels as part of the nutritional assessment, taking into account such factors as age, growth, activity level, medical condition, etc.

Mary's dietitian has determined that she needs 1. 1 gram of protein per kilogram of body weight.

9. CARBOHYDRATE ALLOWANCE. Determine carbohydrate allowance by subtracting protein from the total carbohydrate + protein allowance (Step 7 minus Step 8 above). Carbohydrates are the diet's filler and are always determined last.

Mary's carbohydrate allowance is 25.5–16.5 = 9 grams of carbohydrate daily.

10. MEAL ORDER. Divide the daily fat, protein, and carbohydrate allotments into the desired number of meals and snacks per day. The number of meals will be based on the child's dietary habits and nutritional needs. It is essential that the proper ratio of fat:protein + carbohydrate be maintained at each meal.

Mary's dietitian has decided to give her three meals and no snacks per day:

	DAILY	PER MEAL
Protein	16.5 g	5.5 g
Fat	102.0 g	34.0 g
Carbohydrate	9 g	3.0 g
Calories	1,020	340

Note: This example is simplified for teaching purposes. In reality most four-year-olds would be prescribed one or two snacks in addition to their three meals. The snacks would be in the same ratio (4:1) and the meals reduced by the number of calories in each snack.

11. LIQUIDS. Multiply the child's desirable weight by the value shown on the chart on p. 123 to determine the daily cubic centimeters allotment of liquid. Liquid intake should be spaced throughout the day. Liquids should be noncaloric, such as water or decaffeinated zero-calorie diet drinks. In hot climates the cream may be excluded from the fluid allowance (in other words, liquids may be increased by the volume of the cream in the diet). The liquid allotment may also be set equal to the number of calories in the diet.

Mary, who weighs 15 kg, is allowed $800 + (40 \times 15) = 1,400$ cc of fluid per day, including her allotted cream.

12. DIETARY SUPPLEMENTS. The ketogenic diet is deficient in some nutrients. Multivitamin and mineral supplements are required. In choosing a supplement it is important to consider carbohydrate content. Children who are not medically compromised can usually be adequately supplemented with an over-the-counter, reputable multivitamin and mineral supplement and a separate calcium supplement. Unicap, Centrum, and Poly-Vi-Sol have been used in the past, although the composition of branded products is always subject to change. Most children do well with commercially available supplements, although these have been alleged to lack some micronutrients.

Calorie Levels

There are many standard references for calculating caloric needs for individual children. The following are approximate ranges that have been used at Johns Hopkins for children on the ketogenic diet:

Under 1	75–80 kcal/kg
Ages 1–3	70–75 kcal/kg
Ages 4–6	65–68 kcal/kg
Ages 7–10	55–60 kcal/kg
11 and over	30–40 kcal/kg or less.

Calculating Meal Plans

Calculating the meal plans themselves, in contrast to the diet prescription, is a fairly straightforward procedure. There are currently two different ways of calculating the meal plans: by hand or by computer.

The hand calculation method uses exchange lists and rounded nutritional values for simplicity. This method is cumbersome, time-consuming, and based to a certain extent on nutritional averages. It is, however, the method that was used at Johns Hopkins and elsewhere with much success before the availability of personal computers. It is important that dietitians become familiar with the hand calculation method in order to fully understand the logic of meal planning, and in case a computer is not available in a pinch.

A computer program that greatly simplifies calculation of the meal plans and snacks has been developed. The program may be purchased by calling the Epilepsy Association of Maryland at (410) 828-7700. The program can juggle the nutritional composition of several ingredients in a meal, making meal planning easier. An updated, Y2K-compatible version is available.

The computer program does not replace a professional nutritional assessment. It does not perform the function of a dietitian or nutritionist. It has no judgment or medical knowledge. It cannot monitor a child's health. However, the computer program is a useful mathematical aid.

Because the computer program uses data about the precise nutritional content of specific foods, whereas the hand calculation method relies on averages in order to simplify the math, the computer program may result in slightly different numbers of calories and grams for a given meal than the hand calculation method.

Generic Group A and B vegetables and fruits can be exchanged with both methods of meal calculation. It is easy for parents to switch from one Group A vegetable to another or one 10 percent fruit to another, depending on the child's whims or what is available in the grocery store. The exchange lists assume that there will be some variety in the diet. If the child only likes carrots and grapes—which contain the highest carbohydrate levels on the exchange lists—then she could end up with less than optimal seizure control. In this case the meal plans should be recalculated specifically for carrots and grapes.

The precision of the computer calculations shows the minor differences between the content of, say, broccoli and green beans. For most children these minor differences are of little importance. Therefore, once a meal plan has been calculated by computer, and assuming that the child is doing well on the diet, exchanges may still be made among the foods on the fruit and vegetable exchange lists. If better seizure control is needed, however, it may in some cases be achieved through the use of specific meal plan calculations instead of exchange lists.

With the availability of the computer program, we no longer use meat exchange lists. Meats' fat and carbohydrate contents vary too greatly. The exchange lists are still used with hand calculations.

The dietitian provides parents with a set of basic meal plans before they go home from the hospital. When parents call the dietitian to discuss meal plans, they can refer to these basic meals by title. The basic meal plans are:

1. Meat/fish/poultry, fruit/vegetable, fat, cream.

2. Cheese, fruit/vegetable, fat, cream.

3. Egg, fruit/vegetable, fat, cream.

The meat and cheese should be designated specifically (i.e., chicken, fish, Parmesan) in actual meal plans. When specifics are added, the result will probably be a basic set of six or eight meal plans sent home with the parents from the hospital.

AVERAGE FOOD VALUES FOR HAND CALCULATIONS

	Grams	Protein	Fat	Carbohydrate
36% Cream	100	2. 0	36.0	3.0
Ground Beef	100	24.2	19.1	—
Chicken	100	31.1	2.6	0
Tuna in Water	100	26.8	1.8	0
10% Fruit	100	1.0	0.0	10.0
Group B Vegetable	100	2.0	0.0	7.0

Fat	100	0.0	74.0	—
Egg	100	12.0	12.0	—
Cheese	100	30.0	35.3	—
Cottage Cheese (4%)	100	13.2	4.4	3.5
Cream Cheese	100	6.7	33.3	3.3
Peanut Butter	100	26.0	48.0	22.0

Note: A food contents reference book, such as *Bowes & Church's Food Values,* is helpful for current information on specific foods. As discussed in Chapter 5, cream should be consistent (e.g., 36%), and butter should come in solid, stick form, not whipped or low calorie.

CROSS MULTIPLICATION: THE KEY TO USING THE FOOD LIST

Question: If 100 g 36% cream contains 3.0 g carbohydrate, how much cream contains 2.4 g of carbohydrate?

Step 1: $\dfrac{100}{3} = \dfrac{x}{2.4}$

Step 2: $3x = 240$

Step 3: $x = \dfrac{240}{3} = 80\ g$

Answer: 80 g of 36% cream contains 2.4 g of carbohydrate.

Sample Calculation

1. Jeremy, a 9-year-3-month-old boy, is to be placed on a 4:1 ketogenic diet. His actual weight is 32 kg and his height is 134 cm. According to the standard charts, he is at 50 percent for height but 90 percent for weight. His ideal weight is estimated at 29 kg.

2. The dietitian estimated Jeremy's calorie allotment at 60 calories per kilogram. One of the dietitian's goals was to have Jeremy gradually achieve his ideal weight. Toward this end, Jeremy's total calorie allot-

ment is set by multiplying his *ideal* weight by 60: 29 × 60 = 1,740 calories per day.

3. Each of Jeremy's dietary units will consist of
   4 g fat (× 9 calories per g) = 36 calories
   1 g carbohydrate + protein (× 4 calories per g) = 4 calories
   Total calories per dietary unit = 40 calories

4. Jeremy's dietary units will be determined by dividing his total daily calorie allotment (Step 2) by the calories in each dietary unit: 1,740 calories/40 calories per dietary unit = 43.5 dietary units per day.

5. Jeremy's daily fat allowance is determined by multiplying his dietary units (Step 4 above) by the fat component in his diet ratio (4 in a 4:1 ratio): 43.5 × 4 = 174 g fat.

6. Jeremy's protein needs are at a minimum 1 gram of protein per kilogram of body weight. His ideal weight is 29 kg, so he needs at least 29.0 g protein daily.

7. Jeremy's daily carbohydrate allotment is determined by multiplying his dietary units (Step 4 above) by the 1 in his 4:1 ratio, then subtracting his necessary protein (Step 6 above) from the total: 43.5 – 29 = 14.5 g carbohydrate per day.

Jeremy's complete diet order will read:

	PER DAY	PER MEAL
Protein	29.0 g	9.7 g
Fat	174.0 g	58.0 g
Carbohydrate	14.5 g	4.8 g
Calories	1,740	580

Note: Most children are now given a meal plan that includes one or two snacks, which would diminish the quantity of food in the three main meals. If Jeremy does not lose weight, is not in sufficient ketosis, or turns out to not be as active as originally thought, the caloric amounts will be recalculated during the fine tuning period.

CALCULATING A MEAL

1. Calculate the whipping cream first. Heavy whipping cream should take up no more than half of the carbohydrate allotment in a meal.

2. Calculate the rest of the carbohydrates (fruit or vegetables) by subtracting the carbohydrate contained in the cream from the total carbohydrate allotment.

3. Calculate the remaining protein (chicken, cheese, or egg) by subtracting the protein in the cream and vegetables from the total protein allowance. The total amount of protein may occasionally be off by 0.1 g (over or under) without adverse effect.

4. Calculate the amount of fat to be allowed in the meal by subtracting the fat in the cream and protein from the total fat allowance.

JEREMY'S TUNA SALAD

1. Jeremy is allowed a total of 4.8 g carbohydrate per meal. To use half of this carbohydrate allotment as cream, calculate the amount of 36% cream that contains 2.4 grams of carbohydrate. (See note on cross-multiplication.) Jeremy should eat 80 g of 36% cream, which contains 2.4 g of carbohydrate.

2. For his remaining 2.4 g of carbohydrate, Jeremy can eat 35 g of Group B vegetables, or twice as many Group A vegetables.

3. The 34.3 g Group B vegetables and 80 g 36% cream contain a total of 2.3 g protein (0.68 + 1.6 = 2.3). Jeremy is allowed 9.7 g protein per meal, so he can eat as much tuna as contains 9.7 − 2.3 = 7.4 g protein. Referring to the food values chart, this works out to be 28 g tuna.

4. Jeremy has to eat 58 g fat with each meal. The cream and tuna contain 29.3 g fat, leaving 28.7 g of fat to be mixed in with his tuna fish. Jeremy will get 39 g mayonnaise, which contains 28.9 g fat. (Note that mayonnaise actually has fewer grams of fat than oil does and also contains some protein and carbohydrate. The hand calculation method does not account for these variations).

CALCULATING MEAL PLAN

	Weight	Protein	Fat	Carbohydrate
Tuna	28 g	7.4 g	0.5 g	—
Group B Vegetable	33 g	0.7 g	—	2.3
Fat	39 g	—	28.9 g	—
36% Cream	80 g	1.6 g	28.8 g	2.4 g
Actual Total		9.7 g	58.2 g	4.7 g
Should Be		9.7 g	58.0 g	4.8 g

The 4:1 ketogenic ratio of this menu may be double-checked by adding the grams of protein + carbohydrate in the meal and multiplying by 4. The result should be the amount of fat in the meal, in this case 58 g. Since $(9.7 + 4.8) \times 4 = 58$, the ratio is correct.

NOTES ON JEREMY'S LUNCH

- Jeremy likes his cream frozen in an ice cream ball (slightly whipped), flavored with vanilla and saccharin, and sprinkled with a little cinnamon.

- Jeremy's mom arranges the vegetables in thin-sliced crescents or shoestring sticks around the tuna.

- If Jeremy doesn't like as much mayonnaise with his tuna, some of his fat allowance in the form of oil can be calculated and whipped into the cream one hour after it goes into the freezer. The fats on the exchange list can be used interchangeably—a meal's fat can be provided as all mayonnaise, half mayonnaise and half butter, or the oil may be calculated and mixed with the butter, depending on the child's taste and what makes food sense. In the case of hiding fat in ice cream, oil works nicely because it is liquid and has little flavor.

QUESTIONS AND ANSWERS

Q *How do you add extra ingredients to a meal plan when calculating by hand?*

A Take the tuna salad as an example. Suppose Jeremy wants to sprinkle baking chocolate shavings on his ice cream and bacon bits on the tuna salad. You would add a line for bacon and a line for baking chocolate in your hand or computer calculation. Then choose a small quantity, perhaps 5 grams of bacon and 2 grams of baking chocolate, and fill in the values for protein, fat, and carbohydrate of each. The quantities of other ingredients would then have to be juggled downward until all the columns add up to the proper totals. Bacon, which contains protein and fat, will take away from the meal's tuna and mayonnaise allotment. Baking chocolate, which is primarily fat and carbohydrate with a little protein, will take away from the amount of tomatoes in the meal. As the overall carbohydrate allotment is very small and the nutritive value of chocolate is less than that of vegetables, no more than two grams of chocolate should be used in a meal on the 4:1 ratio. With the accompanying computer program, an additional ingredient may simply be filled in on a blank line, and the other ingredients adjusted until the actual totals match the correctly prescribed ones.

Q *When is it necessary to make calorie adjustments?*

A Weight should be monitored on a weekly basis, and height on a monthly basis. Infants should be weighed and measured accurately at the pediatrician's office about every two weeks. At least during the fine-tuning period, the ketoteam should be informed monthly of a child's height and weight changes and any other relevant information. Once a child is started on the diet, changes in the diet order are usually made in response to her own performance—weight loss or gain, growth in height, seizure control, etc. After a year we evaluate and may make adjustments based on whether she has grown, whether any weight loss or gain has occurred, whether she is still having seizures, and, if so, whether there is any more we can do to control them.

Q   *How often should a child eat on the ketogenic diet?*

A   The number of meals and snacks included in a child's diet should approximate her pre-diet eating habits when possible, the family's schedule, and always take into account her nutritional needs. Infants will need to be given about six bottle feedings a day. Toddlers will probably need three meals and one or two snacks. Older children might need three meals and only one snack. Some children gain better overnight and early morning seizure control by having a bedtime snack. Snacks are sometimes used to test how many extra calories a child who is losing weight needs and whether the extra calories cause any seizure activity problems.

SARAH WAS DOING WELL ON THE DIET, eating three meals and one afternoon snack. Her seizures were virtually gone during the day, but she was still having seizures early every morning. At her follow-up checkup the dietitian learned that Sarah was eating dinner at about 5:30 P.M. going to bed around 7:30, and waking up at 7:00 for breakfast. It seemed that in the 13.5 hours between dinner and breakfast Sarah was running out of fats to make ketones! The dietitian knew that Sarah needed to take in some calories later in the evening. She considered switching dinner to a later hour, but decided it would be easier for the family to move Sarah's snack to bedtime. Once Sarah started eating her snack at bedtime, the early morning seizures disappeared.

Q   *Is it necessary to use half of the carbohydrate allotment as cream?*

A   Using up to half of the carbohydrate allotment as cream is a guideline, not a hard and fast rule. Cream is an easy means to fit a lot of fat into the diet in a way that most children enjoy. If less cream is used, the child will have to eat more mayonnaise, butter, or oil. Some children like to eat fat, some don't. Some children love cream, some don't. As long as the diet makes food sense, there is no need to use half of the carbohydrate allotment as cream.

A DIET ORDER TEST

Lily is 24 months old and weighs 12 kilos. She is 86.5 cm. tall. Both her height and weight are at the 50th percentile. She is going to start on a 4:1 ketogenic diet. What will her diet order read?

1. At age two years, Lily's calorie per kilogram requirement will be approximately 75 calories per kilogram. (As indicated previously, calorie requirements vary with the metabolism and activity level of the child and must be individually assessed.) Her ideal weight is the same as her actual weight, 12 kilograms. So Lily's total calorie allotment is $75 \times 12 = 900$ calories per day.

2. Lily's dietary units will consist of 40 calories each, the standard for a 4:1 diet.

3. Lily's dietary units are determined by dividing her total calorie allotment by the calories in each dietary unit. So she will have $900 / 40 = 22.5$ dietary units per day.

4. Lily's daily fat allowance is determined by multiplying her dietary units (22.5) by the fat component in her ratio (4 in a 4:1 ratio). She will thus be allowed $22.5 \times 4 = 90$ g fat per day.

5. Lily's protein + carbohydrate allotment is 22.5 g per day, determined by multiplying her dietary units (22.5) by the 1 in her 4:1 ratio. As a young, growing child she may need 1.1–1.5 grams of protein/kg. Her weight is 12 kg, so allowing 1.2 grams of protein per kilogram per day makes her protein allotment 14.4 g per day.

6. Lily's daily carbohydrate allotment is determined by subtracting her protein allotment (14.4 g) from the total protein + carbohydrate allowance (22.5 g): $22.5 - 14.4 = 8.1$ g carbohydrate per day.

Lily's complete diet order will read:

	PER DAY	**PER MEAL**
Protein	14.4 g	4.8 g
Fat	90.0 g	30.0 g
Carbohydrate	8.1 g	2.7 g
Calories	900	300

Note: As mentioned previously, most two-year-olds eat one or two snacks in addition to their three meals a day. This example has been simplified for teaching purposes.

MEAL TEST

For dinner, Lily would like to eat grilled chicken with fruit salad and a vanilla popsicle. How would you calculate this meal?

1. Start from the per-meal diet order. Lily is allowed a total of 2.7 g carbohydrate per meal. To use half of this allotment as 36% cream, her popsicle should contain 45 g cream, which will provide 1.35 g carbohydrate.

2. To provide her remaining 1.35 g carbohydrate, she can have 13 g of 10% fruit.

3. The 10% fruit and 36% cream contain a total of 1.03 g protein. Lily's total protein allotment for the meal is 4.8 g, so she can eat as much grilled chicken as will provide 4.8–1.03 = 3.77 g protein. This works out to 12 g chicken.

4. Lily is allowed 30 g of fat in each meal. The chicken and cream contain a total of 16.5 g fat. Lily should eat 17 g of butter or mayonnaise to provide the additional 13.5 g fat allotment.

Lily's dinner plan will read:

CHICKEN CUTLET WITH FRUIT SALAD

	Weight	Protein	Fat	Carbo-hydrate	Calories
36% Cream	45 g	0.9 g	16.2 g	1.4 g	155
Chicken Breast	12 g	3.7 g	0.3 g	—	18
10% Fruit Exchange	13 g	0.1 g	—	1.3 g	6
Butter	17 g	0.1 g	13.8 g	—	125
Actual Total		4.8 g	30.3 g	2.7 g	304
Should Be		4.8 g	30.0 g	2.7 g	300

Notes on Lily's meal: The chicken can be pounded very thin to make it look bigger on the plate. The fruit salad will be pretty if composed of small chunks of water-packed canned peaches and fresh strawberries. Lily thinks it is fun to pick up the chunks with a toothpick. The cream can be diluted with some allotted water, sweetened with saccharin, flavored with four or five drops of vanilla, and frozen in a popsicle mold in advance of the meal. Lily loves butter; she will eat it straight or it can be spread over her chicken. A small leaf of lettuce can be added to the meal for extra crunch.

CHAPTER NINE

LIQUID FORMULAS
AND TUBE FEEDINGS

Children with seizures have all the same nutritional requirements as other children, but some have special needs when it comes to feeding. The ketogenic diet can be modified for all children, whether they are bottle-fed infants, small children making the transition from bottle to soft food, or children with special feeding problems. The ketogenic diet can be formulated in any texture—liquid, soft, solid, or a combination—and can be used even by children who need to be fed by nasogastric or gastrostomy tube.

As discussed in Chapter 8, seizures themselves or the side effects of anticonvulsant medications may affect a child's ability to eat properly. If the seizures are controlled or medications can be reduced with the ketogenic diet, the child may become able to come off soft or liquid diets after a time.

CALCULATING BOTH SOFT AND LIQUID DIETS

The process of calculating the basic diet order, of establishing calorie levels and the grams of fat, protein, and carbohydrate permitted on the ketogenic diet, is the same regardless of the consistency of the food.

The first steps in calculating meal plans of either liquid or soft consistency are the same as those used in calculating a traditional ketogenic diet: follow the calculation process described in Chapter 8. Remember, inactive children may need fewer calories per kilogram than average children. As always, monitor a child's weight closely for the first few months on the diet to make sure calorie levels are set at appropriate levels.

Example: Emily is a 13-month-old girl who has been fed by gastrostomy tube since she was eight months old because of intractable seizures and heavy medication. After conducting a nutritional assessment, Emily's dietitian has determined that she needs to lose weight to achieve optimal ketosis. She'll be started on a 3:1 ratio because she'll be burning her own body fat at a calorie level set to encourage weight loss. The nutritional assessment led the dietitian to prescribe calories at 70/kg and protein at 1.6/kg of desirable body weight.

Emily's age	13 months
Height	29.7" (76 cm), 50th percentile for age
Actual weight	25 lb (11.4 kg), 95th percentile for age
Ideal weight	21.5 lb (9.8 kg), 50th percentile for age
Calories/kg	70
Protein requirement	1.6 g per kg of desirable body weight
Ketogenic ratio	3:1

Using the above numbers in the formula described in Chapter 8, calculate the diet order via the following steps: (Note: numbers are rounded to 0.1 g)

1. Calories: 70 (kcal/kg) × 9.8 (kg ideal weight) = 686 calories per day
2. Dietary unit (see p. 129): 686 (kcal) / 31(kcal/dietary unit) = 22.1 units per day

3. Fat allowance: 3 (as in 3:1) × 22.1 (dietary units) = 66.3 g fat

4. Protein: 1.6 (grams per kg ideal weight) × 9.8 = 15.7 g protein

5. Carbohydrate: 22.1 (protein + carbohydrate) − 15.7 (protein) = 6.4 g carbohydrate

Per the above calculations, Emily's daily diet order, which will be divided into the number of meals or bottles she regularly gets in a 24-hour period, will read:

	Daily
Protein	15.7 g
Fat	66.3 g
Carbohydrate	6.4 g
Calories	686

PREPARING SOFT DIETS

Preparing the ketogenic diet in the form of soft, ground, or strained foods is really a question of texture rather than of theory since the basic technique for formulating a soft-diet meal plan for tube feedings is the same as for solid foods. Commercial baby foods, like all commercially processed foods, should be checked to ensure that there are no added sugars.

WHEN GABRIELLE FIRST STARTED THE KETOGENIC DIET she was unable to swallow liquids without aspirating. She was on high doses of phenobarbital and was having more than a hundred seizures a day. She could eat soft foods, but liquids had to be given through a gastrostomy tube.

Within four months of diet initiation, Gabrielle became almost seizure-free (except when she was sick). The ketoteam started to taper off her phenobarbital. As she came off the medication, Gabrielle not only grew more alert, but also her swallow improved to the point that a swallow study showed she could come off the gastrostomy tube.

PREPARING LIQUID OR TUBE FEEDINGS

The ketogenic diet in liquid form is used primarily for infants and for children who are fed by gastrostomy tube. The process of calculating allotted protein, carbohydrate, and fat is the same for liquid diets as for diets of other consistencies.

Liquid ketogenic diets are most often composed of three ingredients:

- Ross Carbohydrate-free Concentrate (RCF)
  - Soy-based protein, avoids symptoms of cow's milk sensitivities
  - Available through Ross in a concentrated liquid: 13 fluid ounce cans; 12 per case; No. 108
- Microlipid (Mead Johnson)

  A safflower-oil emulsion that mixes easily in solution; made by Mead Johnson
  - Rich source of polyunsaturated fat and high in linoleic acid
  - Available in 120 ml bottles; 24 per case; product code 8884-300400
- Polycose (Glucose Polymers)
  - Source of calories derived solely from carbohydrate
  - Available through Ross in powder form (350 gram cans); 6 per case; No. 746.

Carbohydrate-free multivitamins and minerals, calcium supplements, and sterile water are added to complete the mixture.

FOOD VALUES FOR LIQUID DIET CALCULATION

	Quantity	Protein	Fat	Carbohydrate
RCF Concentrate	100 cc	4.0 g	7.2 g	—
Microlipid	100 cc	—	50.0 g	—
Canola Oil	100 g	—	97.1 g	—
Polycose Powder	100 g	—	—	94.0 g

Because it is emulsified, Microlipid mixes much more easily with the other ingredients than oil would. It is also easier to digest. But Microlipid is also more expensive than corn oil or canola oil. Vegetable oil may be used for larger (older) children or when expense is a factor. MCT oil may also be added to a formula if the dietitian thinks it is needed, i.e., to loosen stools or boost ketosis.

TO SET UP A LIQUID MEAL PLAN

1. *Calculate the amount of RCF needed to satisfy the child's protein requirement by cross-multiplying.*

   Emily's desirable weight is 9.8 kilograms. Her protein requirement is 1.6 g per kilogram of desirable body weight, or $1.6 \times 9.8 = 15.7$ g per day. 100 g of RCF formula contains 4.0 g of protein. Use the following formula:

   $$\frac{100}{4.0} = \frac{X}{15.7} = \frac{100 \times 15.7}{4.0} = 393 \text{ cc}$$

   Emily will need 393 cc RCF concentrate to meet her 15.7 g protein requirement.

2. *Calculate the fat in RCF by cross-multiplying, and calculate enough Microlipid to make up the difference.*

   100 g RCF contains 7.2 g fat. Emily's 393 cc of RCF contains:

   $$\frac{100}{7.2} = \frac{393}{X} = \frac{393 \times 7.2}{100} \text{ or } 28.3 \text{ g fat}$$

   Subtract the 28.3 g fat from the total 66.4 g fat needed ($66.4 - 28.3 = 38.1$). Remaining fat is 38.1 g.

3. *To calculate the Microlipid needed to make up the remaining 37.4 g fat in Emily's diet, cross-multiply.*

   $$\frac{100}{50} = \frac{X}{38.1} = \frac{100 \times 38.1}{50} = X, X = 76.2 \text{ cc Microlipid}$$

4. *Calculate an amount of Polycose powder sufficient to meet Emily's carbohydrate requirement.*

100 g Polycose powder contains 94.0 g carbohydrate. Emily needs 6.8 g Polycose powder to provide her required 6.4 g carbohydrate, determined by the following formula:

$$\frac{100}{94} = \frac{X}{6.4} = \frac{100 \times 6.4}{94} \text{ or } 6.8 \text{ g}$$

5. *The liquid allotment is set at 100 ml per kilogram of desirable body weight, giving Emily 980 ml liquid per day.*

Emily's RCF and Microlipid total 469.2 cc (393 RCF + 76.2 Microlipid). Her water allotment will therefore be 980 – 469.2 = 510.8 cc. This will be rounded to 511 cc.

EMILY'S DAILY FORMULA

	Quantity	Protein	Fat	Carbohydrate
RCF concentrate	393 cc	15.7 g	28.3 g	—
Microlipid	76.2 cc	—	38.1 g	—
Polycose powder	6.8 g	—	—	6.4 g
Sterile water	511 cc	—	—	—
Total	987 cc	15.7 g	66.4 g	6.4 g

Note: In practice this meal would be rounded to the nearest gram for convenience in measuring.

PREPARATION OF KETOGENIC LIQUID FORMULA

1. Measure the RCF concentrate and Microlipid in a graduated cylinder.

2. Weigh the Polycose powder on a gram scale and blend with above ingredients.

3. Add sterile water, reserving 10–15 cc per feeding to flush the tube. Shake or stir.

4. Divide into the number of equal feedings the child will receive in a 24-hour period and refrigerate, or refrigerate full amount and divide into individual portions at feeding time.

5. Bring to room temperature or warm slightly before feeding.

6. Remember to supplement this formula with vitamins and minerals.

Liquid feedings may be given orally or through tubes. They may be given by continuous drip or as periodic feedings. The tubes may be flushed with 10–15 cc of sterile or tap water, but no more than this because of the diet's fluid restrictions.

Some families reserve some of the water for between meal feedings. This is also acceptable as long as the child received the total amount of fluid.

Children on liquid feedings who do not have a swallowing difficulty, such as growing babies, may be "transitioned" to soft foods by gradually substituting the equivalent soft foods for a portion of their bottle feedings.

The liquid ketogenic formula is relatively expensive. Since the ketogenic diet is a therapy rather than a food, WIC programs and many insurance companies will cover its cost. The following sample letter may be of help in communicating the reasons for the diet:

WIC Program
Case Review Services
Re: Ketogenic Diet Therapy

For: _____

DOB: _____

Attention Case Manager:

_____ is a _____-month old boy/girl with a diagnosis of _____ and an intractable seizure disorder. His seizures were occurring _____ times each day despite attempts at seizure control with _____ (name anticonvulsants here).

The ketogenic diet is a high fat, adequate protein, low carbohydrate formula that is individually calculated and prescribed to produce adequate ketosis to suppress the child's seizures. The formula, which is fed by (bottle/gastrostomy tube) is comprised of Ross carbohydrate-free formula, Polycose powder, and Microlipid made by the MeadJohnson company. The formula must be supplemented with multivitamins and minerals in order to be nutritionally complete.

We are requesting that, since these components constitute an anti-epileptic therapy rather than just a nutritional formula, they be covered under your policies.

Thank you for helping _____ to develop as free of seizures and medications as possible.

Sincerely,

KETOGENIC COOKING

CHAPTER TEN

SAMPLE
MEAL
PLANS

Although quantities are limited and smaller than a child is used to, the variety and appeal of food on the ketogenic diet are limited only by your creativity!

- Filet of beef with strawberry cream popsicle
- Eggs Benedict
- Cheese omelette with orange juice
- Shrimp scampi with pumpkin parfait
- Cheesecake

Nearly all the foods your child likes can be transformed into a ketogenic meal. The ketogenic diet can be such a gift—the meals need not be considered a punishment!

AS OFTEN AS POSSIBLE, Michael has something that we are having. If I am making pork chops for us, I cook him one. If we are having tuna

*fish sandwiches, he has tuna fish with mayonnaise wrapped in a leaf of
lettuce. —EH*

Parents should not stray from the basic meal plans in the beginning
for the sake of simplicity and control while learning how to implement
the diet and seeing whether ketosis provides effective seizure control for
their child. When the diet has been proven useful and they are familiar
with its preparation, parents can begin to get more creative with flavorings and new menu plans.

Herbs and spices, lemon juice, soy sauce, baking chocolate, catsup,
and other flavorings all contain carbohydrates. The overall carbohydrate
level in the diet is extremely low, so that catsup calculated into a meal
plan may eliminate your child's fruit or vegetable allotment! Herbs and
spices should be limited to a tiny pinch, and high-carbohydrate flavorings such as catsup or chocolate should only be used occasionally if at all.

Pure vanilla flavoring, up to five drops a meal, has no countable food
value and can be considered "free," which is to say not affecting the
ketogenic balance of the meal. Other pure, carbohydrate-free extracts,
such as almond, lemon, or chocolate, are similarly "free."

IT WAS IMPORTANT TO MY SON *to feel as though he was getting a
dessert. So I always kept a stock of homemade cream popsicles in the
freezer, flavored with vanilla or chocolate (which was calculated into his
meal plans) and a little bit of saccharin. He got one after every dinner.
If he was supposed to have 80 cc of cream and the Tupperware popsicle
molds only held 60 cc, he drank the rest of the cream straight. —CC*

Think of the recipes included in this chapter in terms of entire meal
plans, not as single food items. The ketogenic ratio of food in the diet
must balance within a whole meal, so any food calculated into one part
of the meal affects what can go into other parts.

The menus that follow are examples drawn from the experience of
various parents and are for a "generic" child. Your own meal plans will
take into account your child's calorie level, protein needs, ketogenic
ratio, and individual preferences. When a child has been seizure-free for
a year and your physician allows the ketogenic ratio to be lowered to 3:1,

larger portions of meat, fruit, and vegetables will be allowed to balance against less fat and cream, permitting greater variety and flexibility.

The Ketogenic Cookbook by Dennis and Cynthia Brake (two professional chefs with two children on the ketogenic diet) provides an excellent source of creative ketogenic food ideas. See the beginning of this book for details on how to obtain the book. The Keto Klub newsletter is also a good source of recipes.

> GO TO RESTAURANTS! *Eat together as a family! Enjoy the benefits you get from the diet. Try not to segregate your child or feed her separately from the rest of the family. She will enjoy feeling included. Most kids appreciate the reduction of seizures and freedom from medication more than they covet the food they cannot eat!*

TIPS

Following are tips from parents who have experienced the ketogenic diet:

- Kids don't mind eating the same thing over and over. Find several simple menus that you and your child can agree on, and stick with them. Six to eight menus is probably all you'll need.

- Use a salad plate so the amount of food seems larger.

- Fix a few meals in advance and keep them in the refrigerator in carefully labeled Tupperware containers (breakfast, lunch, etc.) in case you are not there at mealtimes, or for when your child goes to school or to a friend's house. You will build up a huge Tupperware collection.

- Processed meats are a poor source of protein and can affect a child's ability to maintain good ketosis. Minimize use of packaged or processed foods.

- Use the speck of spices that are allowed (but remember they do contain carbohydrate)! A small amount goes a long way toward making the food interesting!

- My son will drink the cream straight down, but I often mix it with sugar-free soda so it will fill him up more.

- Steaming vegetables provides the best nutrition and keeps water weight out of the food.

- Save a couple of favorite meals for extra special times. Use these meals less than once a week so they remain special for times when you are having something your child loves but cannot have, or for times when nothing else sounds good.

- Chopped lettuce with mayonnaise can be a fairly large-looking element of a meal. It really helps fill up the plate, and it helps with bowel movements, too.

- Find places to hide the fat! Oil hides well in applesauce or ice cream. Butter disappears into peanut butter or cream cheese. Tuna, chicken, or egg salad eats up mayonnaise.

- Select dishes that are familiar and resemble your family's normal meals. Try to be creative!

- Don't assume that a zero-calorie powdered drink is OK. Many contain carbohydrates such as maltodextrin. Always read labels carefully!

- Don't mix nasty-tasting medicine or supplements with food. Separate medicines from food as much as possible.

- Do not buy diet foods—use real mayonnaise, butter, eggs, and so on. Diet foods tend to have high water content and extra carbohydrates.

- Counter the small quantity of food with creative shapes and arrangements: slice meat thinly and fan it out. Pound chicken paper thin. Cut carrots into carrot chips, cucumbers into shoestring sticks.

BASIC TECHNIQUES

The recipes in this chapter do not have quantities, as these must be calculated for each individual child. Each recipe is for a whole meal, considered as a unit, because foods in one part of the meal affect what can be included in another part while maintaining the prescribed ketogenic ratio. As a rule, ingredients such as catsup, lemon juice, vinegar, herbs and spices, soy sauce, and baking chocolate are used in very small quantities (such as 2 grams, about 1/8 teaspoon).

Meats should be lean with fat removed. Fish and poultry should be skinless and boneless. This is to ensure that the child's protein allotment will be as close to pure or solid protein as possible.

Cooked foods should be trimmed and weighed on the gram scale after cooking, except in the case of food that is heated only slightly or will not change volume during cooking (such as cheese for melting or eggs). Previously cooked foods do not have to be weighed again after reheating.

Vegetables are most nutritious when steamed. The exchange list in Table 10-1 shows whether a specific vegetable should be weighed raw or cooked.

"What the eye sees, the mind remembers," the old adage goes. But you should never be tempted to "guesstimate" amounts for the sake of speed or efficiency. You may get used to judging how much 25 grams of chicken or 15 grams of applesauce is, but you should always weigh for accuracy. The quantity of each ingredient in these menus varies from child to child, so we have not given exact amounts here. Quantities can be calculated either by hand or by using the computer program in consultation with a doctor or dietitian.

EXCHANGE LISTS

In the hand-calculated ketogenic diet, fruits and vegetables with similar carbohydrate contents have been grouped into lists of items that may be substituted for one another interchangeably (Table 10-1).

When a menu calls for 21 grams of 10 percent fruit, you may choose cantaloupe, orange, strawberry, peach, or any other item from the 10 percent fruit list. Or you may choose to use 14 grams (two-thirds the amount prescribed) of a 15 percent fruit, such as blueberries, pear, or pineapple. Similarly, if a menu calls for 18 grams of a Group B vegetable, you may choose any item or combination of items from the Group B list,

TABLE 10-1

Exchange Lists

FRUIT OR JUICE: FRESH OR CANNED WITHOUT SUGAR

10% (Use amount prescribed)		15% (Use 2/3 amount prescribed)	
Applesauce, Mott's	Papaya	Apple	Kiwi
Cantaloupe	Peach	Apricot	Mango
Grapefruit	Strawberries	Blackberries	Nectarine
Grapes, purple	Tangerine	Blueberries	Pear
Honeydew melon	Watermelon	Figs	Pineapple
Orange		Grapes, green	Raspberries

VEGETABLES: FRESH, CANNED, OR FROZEN
Measure Raw (R) or Cooked (C) as Specified

Group A (Use twice amount prescribed)		Group B (Use amount prescribed)	
Asparagus/C	Radish/R	Beets/C	Kohlrabi/C
Beet greens/C	Rhubarb/R	Broccoli/C	Mushroom/R
Cabbage/C	Sauerkraut/C	Brussels sprouts/C	Mustard greens/C
Celery/C or R	Summer squash/C	Cabbage/R	Okra/C
Chicory/R	Swiss chard/C	Carrots/R or C	Onion/R or C
Cucumbers/R	Tomato/R	Cauliflower/C	Rutabaga/C
Eggplant/C	Tomato juice	Collards/C	Spinach/C
Endive/R	Turnips/C	Dandelion greens/C	Tomato/C
Green pepper/R or C	Turnip greens/C	Green beans/C	Winter squash/C
Poke/C	Watercress/R	Kale/C	

FAT
Unsaturated fats are recommended

Butter	Canola oil	Flaxseed oil	Margarine
Corn oil	Peanut oil	Mayonnaise	Olive oil

including broccoli, mushrooms, or green beans. Or you may choose to use twice that amount, 36 grams, of any Group A vegetable or combination of Group A vegetables, including asparagus, celery, and summer squash.

All the other ingredients in the diet, including meats, fats, and cheeses, should be specified individually in each menu.

Exchange lists allow greater flexibility in using fruits and vegetables. The diet works well with this method, in spite of minor variations in the makeup of each vegetable and fruit. If a child is eating exclusively high-carbohydrate fruits and vegetables such as grapes and carrots, menus should be calculated specifically for these items.

When hand calculation was the norm, meats, fats, and cheeses were also used in generic exchange list form. In spite of significant variations in the content of items on each exchange list, this worked well for some children who could tolerate the resulting fluctuation in diet content. In an effort to provide optimal ketosis for the greatest number of children, and with the more precise computer menu planning now the norm, only fruit and vegetables are now used in generic exchange list form.

"FREE" WAYS TO DRESS UP YOUR CREAM

Ice cream ball	• Dust with a speck of cinnamon or nutmeg
	• Flavor with sweetener and vanilla or calculated baking chocolate
	• Whip in canola oil after one hour of freezing
	• Flavor with sweetener and vanilla or calculated baking chocolate
Whipped parfait	• Layer with calculated berries
	• Sprinkle with a chopped nut
	• Flavor with sweetener and vanilla, lemon, maple, almond, or
	• Serve on top of calculated sugar-free Jell-O
Cream soda	• Pour cream into fruit-flavored sugar-free soda

DON'T FORGET SUPPLEMENTS   The ketogenic diet must be supplemented with a sugarless multivitamin/mineral and a calcium supplement every day.

Note: The following meal plans must be prepared using calculated food amount specified for an individual child.

SCRAMBLED EGG BREAKFAST

Egg   Cream
Butter   Orange juice

Options (The following must be calculated into the meal plan if desired)
   Crisp bacon, ham, or sausage
   Grated cheese in omelets
   Vegetables, fresh fruit, or applesauce instead of juice
   Baking chocolate for cocoa

Beat equal amounts of yolk and white. Cook eggs in a microwave or nonstick pan, which may be sprayed with nonstick vegetable oil. Transfer to scale and weigh, trimming if necessary. Transfer to plate and add any additional butter. For omelets, egg should be cooked flat and thin, then put back in pan, filled with calculated cheese or vegetable/ butter mixture, heated slightly, and scraped thoroughly onto a plate with a small rubber spatula. Garnish plate with calculated crisp bacon and/or grated cheese sprinkles. Dilute cream with water or ice to make it more like milk, or make hot chocolate by melting baking chocolate shavings in cream with sweetener. Your child must consume all the butter on the plate. Drink orange juice or eat fruit last for dessert. If you choose to include bacon or cheese, less egg will be allowed in the meal plan because the protein allotment will be shared.

KETO PANCAKES

Egg

Butter

Sugar-free sweetener

Cottage cheese

Cream

Fresh fruit slices

Beat egg white until stiff. Fold in yolk, cottage cheese, and sweetener. Spray nonstick pan with cooking spray. Pour mixture into pan to form a round disk about 3/4" thick. Cook thoroughly on first side before turning (or the pancake will fall apart). Top with "syrup" made of melted butter mixed with a few drops of sweetener and carbohydrate-free pure maple flavoring. Serve with fruit slices on the side.

WESTERN OMELETTE

Egg

Mayonnaise

Cream

Dill, basil, salt, pepper

Tomato

Green pepper

Onion

Scramble egg and weigh. Add a little of allotted cream and scramble again. Pour into heated pan coated with vegetable cooking spray. Chop vegetables. Sprinkle with pinch of spices. Mix with mayonnaise. Spread vegetable/mayonnaise mixture on egg. Then flip top over to make omelette and cook a few more minutes until done. This omelette may also be made in a sandwich machine by pouring half of the egg on the grid, spreading the vegetable mixture on top, then adding the other half of the egg and closing the machine until done.

EASY APPLE-SAUSAGE BAKE

Unsweetened applesauce

Butter

Sweetener, vanilla

Bob Evans sausage link

Cream

Speck of cinnamon

Broil sausage link under medium flame until brown, boil until done, or sauté in frying pan. Drain on paper towel. Weigh and trim. Meanwhile, place applesauce in small ovenproof container. Mix in brown sugar substitute or sweetener, top with butter, and place under broiler. Whip cream until it thickens, add a few drops of vanilla and sweetener, and continue beating until stiff. When applesauce is warm and butter is melted, top with whipped cream and dust with cinnamon. Serve with sausage.

APPLESAUCE is a great place to hide fat. As much as equal parts fat to applesauce will blend in and taste good. Add 1/4 grain of saccharin dissolved in warm water or a dash of liquid sweetener to unsweetened applesauce and dust with a speck of cinnamon before serving. May be served warm or at room temperature.

STRAWBERRY CHOCOLATE CHIP ICE CREAM WITH BACON

(Christopher's favorite breakfast)

Bacon	Strawberries
Cream	Canola oil
Vanilla, sweetener	Baking chocolate

Ice cream can be made up to a week beforehand: Dissolve saccharin tablet in 1/2 teaspoon of warm water. Add to cream in a small Pyrex dish. Flavor with vanilla to taste, baking chocolate shavings, and sliced fresh strawberries. Freeze about 1 hour, or until ice begins to form. Remove from freezer. Stir in canola oil quickly and return to freezer. Unmold and serve in a small bowl with crisp bacon on the side.

VARY THE FRUIT (peach, raspberry), omit the chocolate or melt it into cream, or add pure maple extract and chopped nuts for variety. Omitting chocolate or substituting chopped nuts for fruit has to be calculated, of course. Cream may be whipped before freezing.

QUICHE LORRAINE (CUSTARD WITH BACON)

Egg   Cream
Bacon   Orange

Heat cream to scald. Do not boil. Stir beaten egg into cream. Stir in crumbled bacon. Pour mixture into a custard cup. Place in a pan of water. Microwave or bake at 350° until done (about 25 minutes, or until a silver knife inserted in the middle comes out clean). Serve in the custard cup in the middle of a small plate, with thin orange slices arranged around the cup in the shape of a flower.

TUNA SALAD PLATE

Tuna   Mayonnaise
Cream   Sugar-free Jell-O
Sour cream   Parmesan cheese
Baking chocolate   Cucumber, tomato, celery, lettuce

Mix mayonnaise and tuna; arrange in center of plate. Stir together sour cream and Parmesan; mix with chopped lettuce and arrange around tuna. Garnish plate with cucumbers and tomatoes. For dessert, sugar-free Jell-O topped with sweetened vanilla whipped cream, sprinkled with baking chocolate shavings.

HARD-BOILED EGG, cubed chicken or turkey, or baby shrimps may be substituted for the tuna. These salads are easy to prepare in advance, making them ideal travel or school meals.

PEANUT BUTTER CELERY SNACKS

Celery strips   Peanut butter
Butter

Wash thin celery ribs. Peel to remove any strings. Slice off bottom for better stability. Weigh and trim. Combine peanut butter with half of allotted butter. Mix thoroughly. Fill the cavity of celery ribs with peanut butter-butter mixture. Cut into 3-inch pieces. Note: this menu does not have enough protein to be used as a full meal.

IN THE ABSENCE OF TOAST, it's nice to have something crispy that holds a shape, like celery or cucumber boats. —JS

CHEF'S SALAD WITH MAPLE WALNUT WHIP

American cheese	Ham and/or turkey
Lettuce, olive	Oil
Vinegar	Cucumber, tomato, mushroom, carrot
Cream	Crushed walnut
Pure maple extract, sweetener	

Combine chopped lettuce, sliced mushrooms, and carrots in a bowl. Arrange tomato and cucumber slices, olive, and strips of cheese, ham, and/or turkey on top. Shake or beat with a fork the oil and vinegar, a speck of salt and pepper, and a few flakes of oregano in a jar with a tight lid (mayonnaise may be substituted for some of the oil for thicker consistency). Pour over salad. Sprinkle a few parsley flakes and a dash of Accent over all. For dessert: whip cream until thick. Add 3 or 4 drops of pure maple extract and a few drops of sweetener, and continue whipping until stiff. (Several grams vegetable oil may also be whipped into cream if there is too much oil for the salad.) Heap into a parfait dish. Sprinkle with crushed walnuts and serve. Or use butterscotch extract and chopped pecans instead for Butterscotch Fluff.

SPINACH SALAD

Hard-boiled egg	Spinach
Crisp bacon	Mushroom, carrot, red onion
Olive oil, vinegar	Dried mustard, garlic salt
Cream	Butter
Vanilla, sweetener	

Wash spinach, chop coarsely, place in bowl. Sprinkle with chopped red onion, sliced mushroom, and carrot. Shake oil and vinegar together in a jar with a speck of dried mustard, garlic salt, and pepper. Pour over salad. Sprinkle with crumbled crisp bacon and chopped egg (equal parts white and yolk). Serve with vanilla shake or popsicle.

At one point my son started gaining weight and I couldn't figure out why. Then Mrs. Kelly and I reviewed everything I was doing. I had started hiding a lot of fat in ice cream in the form of canola oil because my son had gotten tired of eating so much butter on top of everything. But I was measuring the oil, like the cream and juice, by volume. Lighter liquids are approximately equal when measured either by weight or volume. But because it is so heavy, oil has to be measured on a gram scale. When I started measuring the canola oil on the gram scale instead of in the graduated cylinder, the weight gain stopped.—JS

DEVILED EGG WITH BERRY PARFAIT

Hard-boiled egg	Carrots, celery, onion
Butter, mayonnaise	Dried mustard, paprika
Grated lemon rind	Lettuce
Cream	Vanilla, sweetener, chocolate

Cut egg in half lengthwise and weigh equal amounts of white and yolk. Mix yolk thoroughly with mayonnaise, a few grams melted butter, a speck of dried mustard, chopped celery, and onion. Spoon yolk mixture back into the egg white. Sprinkle with salt and pepper. Dust with paprika. Serve on a plate with chopped lettuce mixed with mayonnaise and vinegar. For dessert, add vanilla and sweetener to cream and whip until stiff. Alternate whipped cream in a parfait dish with layers of sliced raspberries or strawberries.

WEIGH ALL GROUP A vegetables together, and weigh all Group B vegetables together at one time.

SHRIMP SCAMPI

Shrimp	Butter
Cream	Spinach
Garlic salt	

Steam shrimp and weigh. Melt butter in dish with shrimp. Add pinch of garlic salt. Steamed chopped spinach. Pat dry. Stir in some of cream if desired. Fix cream for beverage or dessert as desired.

GRILLED SALMON WITH FRESH TOMATO SALSA*

Salmon	Tomato
Garlic	Onion
Green bell pepper	Black olives
Cilantro	Olive oil
Cream	

Spray pan with Pam; heat; season salmon with speck of salt and pepper; sear over medium to high heat until done but not dry. Remove salmon from the pan and pat dry before weighing. Meanwhile, dice tomatoes, garlic, onion, and green pepper very fine. Mix with cilantro-flavored oil (place 1 g cilantro in an ounce of oil, let sit for three days, strain) and a speck of sea salt and pepper. Let sit for a few hours so flavors can come together. Serve salmon topped with salsa, and banana flavored ice cream.

*Reproduced with permission from *The Ketogenic Cookbook* by Dennis and Cynthia Brake.

CHICKEN SOUP AND CUSTARD

Egg	Diced chicken
Cream	Granulated bouillon
Salt (a speck)	Carrots, celery, lettuce
Saccharin (1/8 grain)	Butter, mayonnaise

Custard: Scald 3 parts cream to 1 part water. Combine with 2 parts beaten egg, salt, saccharin, and vanilla. Pour into a cup and bake in a shallow pan of water 25 minutes at 350° or until done (knife inserted in center will come out clean).

Soup: Dissolve bouillon cube in 1/2 cup hot water. Add enough chicken to make up the protein left over from the egg (if any), and carrots and celery to fill the carbohydrate allotment. Melt a little butter into the soup, and spread the rest of the fat as mayonnaise on lettuce. Drink any leftover cream as beverage.

IN THE CHICKEN SOUP RECIPE, the carrots can also be made into sticks and eaten dipped in mayonnaise instead of being diced into the soup.

CREAM OF TOMATO SOUP WITH GRILLED SWORDFISH

Tomato sauce	Celery, onion
Cream	Fresh swordfish
Speck of tarragon, salt, pepper	Mayonnaise, oil
Lettuce leaf	Chocolate extract, sweetener

Sauté celery and onion in about 5 grams butter. Add tomato sauce. Add a speck each of tarragon, salt, and pepper. Add half of cream allotment and water to thin to desired consistency. Stir until smooth and heat until warm. Meanwhile grill or broil seasoned swordfish, trim and weigh. Serve with a salad of chopped lettuce mixed with mayonnaise. For dessert, put chocolate extract drops into rest of cream and pour into bowl of ice cream scoop. Chill for 1 hour. Stir in canola oil quickly and return to freezer. Freeze until hard.

FOR A VARIETY OF CREAM SOUPS, asparagus, broccoli, or spinach may be substituted for the tomato.

TREATS

BUTTER LOLLIPOPS

Soften butter. Add a tiny drop of vanilla and carbohydrate-free sweetener. Press into candy molds. Add lollipop sticks and freeze one hour or
overnight. Calculate weight not including the sticks, and serve with
meals or snacks.

MACAROON COOKIES

2 egg whites
1/2 tsp. cream of tartar
1/2 package sugar-free Jell-O

Beat egg white until stiff. Add cream of tartar and dry Jell-O. Drop
on aluminum foil sprayed lightly with nonstick cooking spray. Bake
at 325° for 6 to 8 minutes, until brown. Cool before eating. Makes 20
cookies. One serving of two cookies contains 1.0 g protein, 0 g fat, 0.1 g
carbohydrate.

MACADAMIA BUTTERCRUNCH

Chopped macadamia nuts   Butter

Macadamia nuts are naturally in a 3:1 ratio. Add enough butter to bring
them to a 4:1 ratio. This snack is good for school kids and is easy to bring
along on trips.

EGGS BENEDICT*

Beaten egg   Cream
Grated cheddar cheese   Butter
Canadian bacon   Cantaloupe
Vanilla, sweetener

Scramble eggs and weigh. Place on top of heated Canadian bacon. Top with butter and cheese. Melt in broiler or microwave. Serve with cantaloupe. In a blender, blend cream with a few drops of vanilla and sweetener and two ice cubes until ice is ground into a frothy vanilla shake.

---

*Reproduced with permission from *The Ketogenic Cookbook* by Dennis and Cynthia Brake.

"SPAGHETTI"

Spaghetti squash	Cream
Parmesan cheese	Butter
Lettuce	Mayonnaise
Hunt's tomato sauce	Ground beef or ground turkey

Boil squash (raw squash may be frozen in individual portions in advance). Drain well and weigh. Cook and weigh ground meat, and sprinkle on squash. Melt butter with tomato sauce and some or all of cream. Pour on top. Sprinkle grated cheese plus a speck of pepper and oregano if desired. Mix chopped lettuce with mayonnaise for a salad. Pour any remaining cream in a zero-calorie flavored soda and whip lightly for dessert.

> EVEN THE SMALLEST SPRINKLE of Parmesan cheese has to be calculated into the diet. Meatballs can be frozen for later use.

HOT DOG AND CATSUP

Hebrew National hot dog	Butter
Cream cheese	Zucchini or asparagus
Heavy cream	Lettuce
Catsup	Baking chocolate
Vanilla, sweetener	Sugar-free Jell-O

Boil hot dog, drain, weigh. Mix catsup with mayonnaise to make special sauce. Cut into thin slices; dab sauce on each slice. Arrange on a small plate. Spread cream cheese (with some of the butter mixed in if desired) on lettuce. Steam vegetables; pat dry. For dessert (make in advance) add a few drops flavoring, a little sweetener, and cream to the sugar-free Jell-O. Allow to set. Or whip cream into sweetened Jell-O and freeze in the bowl of an ice cream scoop. This is keto sherbet.

WITH COMMERCIAL PRODUCTS   such as hot dogs, the brand must always be specified. Brands of hot dog other than Hebrew National may be used in this recipe if calculations are based on accurate information about the specified brand. Jell-O desserts are often calculated into hot dog meals to raise the protein.

BROILED STEAK WITH BROCCOLI

Steak	Broccoli
Cream	Mayonnaise
Butter	

Broil steak to medium rare. Weigh. Steam broccoli. Melt butter, blend with mayonnaise, pour over broccoli. Serve with cream poured into orange flavored zero-calorie soda.

PEPPER STEAK STIR FRY AND BAVARIAN CREAM

Thin-sliced beef	Green pepper
Onions	Mushrooms
Vanilla	Sweetener
Lettuce	Gelatin
Baking chocolate	Butter, oil
Dash of soy sauce	

Bavarian cream: Swell 2 grams of gelatin with 2 tablespoons cold water. Add 2 grams baking chocolate and a little of allotted butter. Place over warm water until baking chocolate, butter, and gelatin are melted. Stir in 1/4 grain saccharin, a few drops vanilla, and cream. Pour into mold and freeze until hardened.

Stir fry: Heat oil equal to remaining fat allotment after butter used in Bavarian cream (some fat may be reserved for use as oil or mayonnaise in salad dressing). Sauté onions, mushrooms, and green pepper. Season with a speck of salt, pepper, and a dash of soy sauce. Cook beef separately in broiler or microwave. Weigh. Add to vegetables and serve. On the side, serve a chopped lettuce leaf with any remaining oil or mayonnaise for dressing.

> IN THE BAVARIAN CREAM MEAL, total fat allotment is divided into three dishes. You can decide how much butter to melt into the Bavarian cream, how much oil to use with the stir fry, and how much oil or mayonnaise to use as salad dressing as long as all fats add up to the correct total.

BURGER WITH "POTATO SALAD"

Ground beef	Zucchini
Catsup	Mayonnaise, oil
Salt, pepper	Oregano
Cream	Lettuce
Vanilla, sweetener	Sugar-free Jell-O

Flatten the ground beef into a 1/4-inch thick burger. Heat a nonstick skillet with a few drops of the allotted oil or cooking spray. Sauté the burger 1 to 1-1/2 minutes on each side. Weigh the sautéed burger and trim. Meanwhile, measure the catsup and beat in an equal amount of oil. Steam zucchini. Weigh and cut into 1/2-inch cubes. Mix the zucchini with mayonnaise, oregano, and a pinch of salt and pepper. Arrange the beef on a lettuce leaf. Spread catsup mixture on steak. For dessert, top sugar-free Jell-O with whipped sweetened vanilla cream.

I BOUGHT THE KIND OF BLENDER that's a wand you can stick right into a tall glass. You just rinse the wand off in the sink after you use it. That way I don't have to wash the whole blender every time. —FD

"PIZZA"

Egg	Olive oil
Tomato puree	Mozzarella cheese
Cream	Pepperoni or ground beef
Lettuce	Speck of oregano
Vanilla, sweetener	

Beat egg with cream. Pour into heated nonstick pan. Spread thinly. Turn heat to low and let sit until hardened. Mix olive oil with tomato sauce; spread on egg crust. Sprinkle with a speck of oregano. Cover with grated cheese. Top with pepperoni or ground beef. Broil until melted. Serve with diluted cream shake. Note: A thin slice of eggplant, broiled, can serve as crust for alternative recipe.

A THIN TOMATO SLICE may be substituted for the egg-cream or eggplant pizza crust. Triangular slices of cheese can also make a fun pretend pizza!

BROILED FISH WITH TARTAR SAUCE

Flounder or other fish	Butternut squash
Lettuce	Sugar-free Jell-O
Tartar sauce	Butter, mayonnaise
Cream	Accent, pepper

Broil the fish about 5 minutes or until flaky. Season with a speck of Accent and pepper. Spread with measured tartar sauce. Bake butternut squash or cook frozen puree. Melt butter into squash puree. Arrange flounder on a small plate with squash and chopped lettuce with mayonnaise. Serve sugar-free Jell-O topped with whipped cream for dessert.

I DON'T COOK WITH BUTTER as the allowed fat. Since the fat is his body fuel, I want him to get as much as possible. When you cook with butter, you can easily lose some of it in the pan. I usually just spray the pan with non-stick aerosol spray, cook the food, and add the butter while it's hot. —EH

CHICKEN FINGERS AND COLE SLAW

Chicken breast	Scallion
Cream	Cabbage, carrot
Mayonnaise	Butter
Vanilla, sweetener	

Heat a few drops oil in a nonstick skillet. Sauté chicken breast at medium-high heat for about 3 minutes per side or until lightly browned. Remove chicken from heat; weigh and trim. Turn heat off. Add butter (1/3 of fat allotment) to skillet. Add a dash of mustard, tarragon, and garlic salt. Stir until butter is melted. Remove skillet from heat. Cut chicken breast into thin strips or very thin slices and fan out on a small plate. Pour butter sauce over chicken. Meanwhile, chop cabbage (red or green) with a little grated carrot, thinly sliced scallion, and a leaf of lettuce. Mix mayonnaise (2/3 of fat allotment) with a couple of grams of vinegar. Stir in cabbage mixture. Sprinkle with salt and pepper. Serve with frozen vanilla-flavored cream ball.

BEEF STEW

Roast beef	Pearl onions
Cabbage	Cherry tomatoes
Turnips	Cream
Baking chocolate	Sweetener

Steam cabbage, turnip, and onion until tender. Place them in a small, nonstick pot (such as a one-cup Pyrex) with the roast beef and 1/4 cup water. Add butter and sprinkle with a speck of salt and pepper. Simmer 15 minutes. For thicker sauce, mash some turnip into the liquid. Place cherry tomato halves around a small plate and spoon stew in center. Serve with chocolate ice cream.

CHICKEN CUTLET WITH APPLE À LA MODE

Chicken	Butter/Mayonnaise
Lettuce	Cream
Cinnamon	Saccharin
Apple slice	

Chicken cutlet: Pound the chicken very thin between sheets of waxed paper. Grill or pan fry for 1 minute on each side. Sprinkle with a speck of seasoned salt or salt and pepper, and dot with some of allotted butter if desired. Spread lettuce leaf with butter or mayonnaise, roll into a pinwheel, cut in half, and arrange on small plate with chicken.

Apple à la mode: Cut center slice from a small apple. Leave skin on, remove core, and weigh. Sauté in remaining butter in a small skillet until soft. Dust with a speck of cinnamon. Place apple slice in an ice cream dish and top with a ball of sweetened vanilla frozen cream. Pour any cinnamon butter remaining in skillet on top of ice cream. (*Optional:* Serve with Shasta red apple diet drink.)

CHICKEN WITH MASHED TURNIPS

Chicken breast	Turnips
Butter	Cream

Broil chicken breast or sauté it in a nonstick skillet with a few drops of oil. Season chicken with a few flakes of tarragon or oregano if desired. Boil turnips until soft. Mash with butter. Season with salt and pepper. Serve with a chopped lettuce leaf and diluted cream.

CHRIS LOVED MASHED BUTTERED TURNIPS *because they reminded him of potatoes, and he loved potatoes even though he couldn't have them.—JS*

LAMB WITH CUCUMBER AND TOMATO SALAD

Lamb chop	Cucumber
Mayonnaise	Tomato
Vinegar	Baking chocolate
Olive oil	Cream

Broil lamb chop 4 minutes on each side. Season with a speck of pepper and Accent or rosemary if desired. Trim off fat and weigh lamb. Slice meat thinly and fan out on plate. Cut cucumber and tomato into 1/2-inch cubes. Combine vinegar and olive oil and pour over cucumber-tomato salad. Serve on a chopped or rolled lettuce leaf spread with mayonnaise and a chocolate popsicle for dessert.

"TACOS"

Ground beef	Chopped tomato
Lettuce	Grated cheese or sour cream
Cream	Speck of chili powder

Cook beef in nonstick pan. Weigh. Dust beef with a speck of chili powder. Roll beef, tomato, and cheese or sour cream in lettuce leaf. Pour cream into up to 120 grams of orange diet soda for a dessert drink.

EVERY WEEKEND I WOULD MAKE 21 ICE CREAM SERVINGS. My son didn't like much fat in his meals, so I hid almost all of it in the ice cream, which he loved and ate with every meal. I had to plan my menus in advance so I would know how much fat I had to hide in the ice cream for each meal. Mostly I used canola oil, which whips into the cream beautifully just before it freezes. There would be different quantities of oil whipped in with the cream, depending on each menu. Sometimes I would choose a menu with fruit and make strawberry ice cream. I had to label the ice cream very carefully as to which day and which meal they were made for. —JS

JELL-O MOLD

Sugar-free Jell-O	Cottage cheese
Cream cheese	Sour cream
Cream	Butter

Make Jell-O ahead of time and start to cool in the refrigerator. Meanwhile, whip cream. Whip in softened cream cheese, sour cream, and butter. Add 1/4 gram saccharin if desired. Stir into cool liquid Jell-O and let harden. Note: This menu is helpful for children who do not chew well. Every bite is ketogenic, which means it can also be used for children during illness.

BECAUSE CREAM contains so much fat, the more cream you use the less oil, mayonnaise, and butter you will have to fit into the rest of the menu. But if your child doesn't mind eating a lot of mayonnaise or butter, you can use less cream and fill out the carbohydrate allotment with more vegetables or fruit.

CHEESECAKE: A BIRTHDAY MEAL!

Egg	Butter
Cottage cheese	Cream
Sour cream	Fruit
Cream cheese	Vanilla, sweetener

Mix together all ingredients except fruit. Add vanilla to taste and 1/2 grain of saccharin dissolved in 1/2 teaspoon of warm water or liquid sweetener to taste. Bake in small, greased Pyrex dish at 350° for 25 minutes or until light golden on top. Cool. Arrange fruit slices on top—sliced strawberries, pineapple, or peach. Makes a whole meal! Save a bit of cream to whip and pile on top for extra excitement.

A CHEESECAKE MEAL is easy to carry to school in its container for special occasions, such as when other kids are eating cake to celebrate a birthday. Cheesecake also provides a ketogenic ratio in every bite, so it is useful for children who cannot eat a full meal (e.g., when recovering from an illness).

THANKSGIVING CUSTARD

Turkey breast	Green beans
Turnip	Canned pumpkin
Cream	Beaten egg
Butter	Speck of cinnamon
Sweetener	

Weigh cooked turkey breast. Mash turnip with butter. Top green beans and/or turkey with rest of butter. Dessert: Whip egg, cream, canned pumpkin, dash of cinnamon, and sweetener. Bake at 325° in Pyrex dish. Note: Cranberry sauce may be calculated into the menu, replacing both green beans and turnip.

KETOGENIC EGGNOG

Cream	Egg
Vanilla	Saccharin

Beat egg slightly. Weigh. Dissolve saccharin in 1 teaspoon or more water. Add to cream. Combine egg, cream, vanilla, and sweetener to taste. Whip lightly if desired. Sprinkle with nutmeg. Use as travel meal or for an occasional snack. When put in the microwave, eggnog turns into a loose scrambled egg consistency.

LIKE THE CHEESECAKE, frozen eggnog in a margarine tub makes a great birthday party food. Try decorating top with fruit (strawberries, cherries). Wrap the margarine tub in colored foil and take it to school for birthday parties.

QUESTIONS ABOUT PREPARING THE DIET

Q   *Is it good to use high-fat meats to increase the fat content of the diet?*

A   Protein is very important for your child's growth. The protein portion of the diet should therefore be close to pure. Meat should be lean, trimmed of fat. Chicken and fish should be without skin. Cooked fat may be trimmed off and measured separately as part of the fat allotment for the meal. High-fat processed meats such as sausage and bologna should be calculated in the menu according to the manufacturer's contents.

Q   *What if some of the food sticks to the pan?*

A   Use nonstick pans and nonstick spray, and scrape out as much as possible with a small rubber spatula. Cook at low temperatures to avoid burning. Better yet, prepare food using nonstick methods: bake or broil meats, microwave eggs, steam vegetables. Remember that the allotted weights are for cooked food unless otherwise indicated, so until you are experienced with the difference between raw and cooked weights, your meats and vegetables or fruits should be prepared and cooked separately and then assembled with fats at the end.

Q   *Should I try to use margarine instead of butter?*

A   We recommend that you use as many unsaturated fats as possible, such as canola, safflower, flaxseed, or olive oil, or margarine made from canola oil. However, no research exists on the effect of a diet comprised of 90 percent fat, whether saturated or unsaturated. No data indicate that the ketogenic diet, despite its high fat content, leads to heart disease or atherosclerosis later in life.

Q   *My child is too disabled to care much what she eats, so I just want the simplest menu to prepare. What is easiest?*

A   The simplest ketogenic menu planning involves using the four main food groups of the diet without embellishment:

Protein (meat, fish, chicken, cheese, egg)

Carbohydrate (fruit or vegetable)

Fat (butter, margarine, mayonnaise, oil)

Cream

It takes very little time to broil a bit of meat or chicken, steam a piece of broccoli or cut up a tomato, put butter on the chicken or mayonnaise on the broccoli, and serve with a cup of cream diluted with ice and water. For a softer consistency, try fruit-topped cheesecake or custard with bacon and cooked vegetables.

Q *What if the family has to travel or I don't have time to prepare a meal?*

A The eggnog recipe that you receive from your dietitian is a very good emergency or convenience food on the ketogenic diet. Chopped macadamia nuts mixed with butter can also be eaten for an occasional meal. You should not use these meals too often in the diet, but they can tide you over in a pinch. When traveling, take up to two days' meals ahead of time and take them along in a portable cooler. Ask restaurants to microwave them for you if appropriate. Tuna salad with sliced vegetables such as celery, cucumbers, or carrots is especially mobile. See Chapter 6 for further details.

Q *Can I decrease the amount of cream and use more fat in a given menu?*

A Cream is an easy, palatable way to get a lot of fat into the diet. If desired, however, the diet can be calculated with little or no cream. The challenge will be to find ways to make a large quantity of fats or oils palatable.

RECENT ADVANCES

CHAPTER ELEVEN

STUDIES AND NEW DATA

Despite the ongoing development of new anticonvulsant medications, many children continue to have difficult-to-control seizures. The reawakening of interest in the diet has begun to generate new studies of the efficacy and consequences of the diet. Only through such studies will it be possible to truly compare the benefits and the side effects of the ketogenic diet with those of the newer anticonvulsant medications.

On the benefits side, our 1998 evaluation of 150 consecutive children (see Table 3-4) who averaged more than 600 seizures per month before starting the diet *and* had failed more than six anticonvulsants documented that:

- Seven percent of those starting the diet became seizure-free.

- Twenty-seven percent of all those children starting the diet had at least a 90 percent decrease in their seizure frequency. Many of these children had had only one or a few seizures (usually associated with illness) during the month before their one-year assessment.

- Half of all of the children who started on the diet had had better than a 50 percent decrease in their seizures after one year, and more than half of those who tried the diet remained on it for more than one year.

- More than half of the children who stayed on the diet for one year had stopped all of their medications. Many others had decreased the number or amounts of medications.

These figures are similar to the results of studies done in prior decades and are better than any of the studies done with new anticonvulsant medications.

STUDIES IN PROGRESS

Critics sometimes note that the ketogenic diet has never been studied in a blinded, controlled study. Such a study is currently in progress.

In evaluating the effectiveness of the ketogenic diet for the management of the atonic-myoclonic seizures of the Lennox-Gastaut syndrome, we found that the frequency of these "drop" seizures often dramatically decreased during or after the fasting phase of the diet. The meticulous, computerized records of a child's "drop" seizures kept by one family are shown in Figure 11-1.

As can be seen, the child documented in Figure 11-1 had 125 to 350 seizures per week. As the diet was initiated, the records documented a dramatic drop in seizures. (Incidentally, the child has remained seizure-free and medication-free over the following two years and remains seizure-free after being tapered from the diet.) Similar results in other patients are shown in Figure 11-2. This figure shows the rapid decrease in atonic-drop seizures occurring as many patients are fasted and the diet initiated. This and many similar observations piqued our interest in the possibility of studying the efficacy of the diet in a short-term cross-over study.

Our hypothesis was that if the ketogenic diet was effective in decreasing the "drop" seizures because of the ketosis produced, and if we could quickly negate that ketosis with glucose and reinitiate it with fasting,

FIGURE 11-1

Decrease in "drop" seizures in one patient with fasting and initiation of the ketogenic diet.

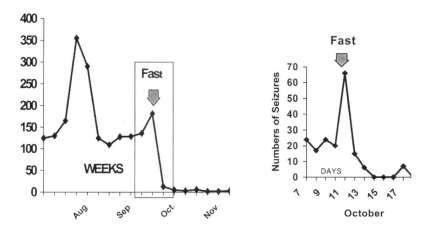

FIGURE 11-2

Seizure response to ketogenic diet.

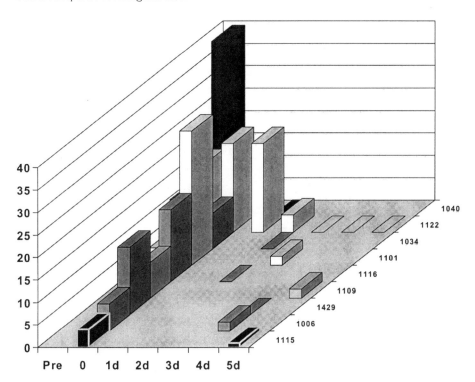

then it would be possible to do a short-term cross-over study of the effectiveness of the diet.

A critical element of such a study would be the objective confirmation of the parental seizure reports by a 24-hour EEG quantifying the electroclinical events (seizures) reported by the parents.

As shown in Figure 11-3, electrical seizures are far more frequent during the nighttime hours, when parents are less likely to see and report them. Thus the parental reports of these "drop" seizures usually substantially underreport their true incidence. Also note the dramatic decrease in measured seizures (dark bars) after the institution of the ketogenic diet.

Preliminary evidence of the rapid effect of the diet on the "drop" seizures of the Lennox-Gastaut syndrome, and the rapid ability to negate the ketosis with the administration of glucose, made it feasible to assess—in a randomized, blinded, cross-over, placebo-controlled fashion—the effectiveness of the ketogenic diet in reducing the number of atonic-myoclonic seizures in children with the Lennox-Gastaut syndrome. The protocol is shown in Figure 11-4.

Children with the Lennox-Gastaut syndrome who had more than 20 parent-reported "drop" seizures each day would be eligible for the study. If the 24-hour EEG confirmed more than 20 seizures, the child would begin fasting for 36 hours. On Day 3 the child would start one-third of the diet eggnog, with two-thirds on the fourth day and the full diet on the fifth day. A repeat 24-hour EEG would document the seizure frequency, and the child would again be fasted and the diet reinitiated. At the end of the second phase, the Digitrace EEG would again be repeated. During one phase of the diet the child would drink liquid containing glucose, thus negating the effects of the diet. During the other phase the liquid would be sweetened with saccharin, which would not negate the ketogenic effects of the diet. No one involved with the child would know which phase contained glucose. This study, funded by the NIH, is in progress as of this writing. If the effectiveness of the diet is documented in such a study, it is likely to lead to its more widespread acceptance and use in appropriate populations.

FIGURE 11-3
Digitrace recordings pre- and post-diet initiation. Bursts of spike and slow waves were of much shorter duration post-diet.

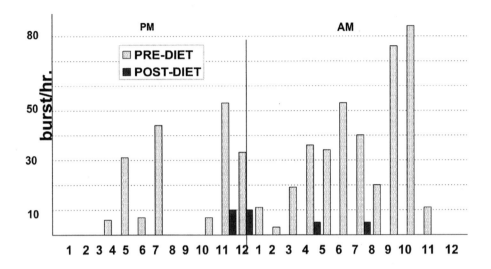

FIGURE 11-4
Ketogenic diet "drop" seizure protocol.

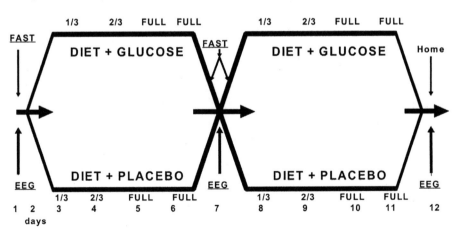

SIDE EFFECTS CURRENTLY UNDER STUDY

Is the ketogenic diet nutritionally adequate? Does it impair growth? Doesn't eating all that fat make the children obese? These are some of the questions we frequently hear.

NUTRITION: The ketogenic diet is nutritionally adequate EXCEPT that it requires supplementation with calcium and with fat-soluble vitamins. In some children hair may begin to fall out or may become coarse and reddish. This may be due to lack of minerals but has not been adequately studied. We supplement those children with a carbohydrate-free mineral supplement.

GROWTH: Ongoing studies indicate that most children grow normally on the ketogenic diet. Indeed, some profoundly handicapped children grow at a faster rate when their nutrition is carefully monitored on the diet and when they are less sedated by medications. A few children do not seem to have grown on the diet at Johns Hopkins. Whether this lack of growth is caused by the diet or is part of their underlying problem remains unclear. When these children return to a normal diet, they will be monitored to see if a growth spurt occurs.

WEIGHT GAIN: The diet is initially calculated to be calorically adequate to bring the child close to his or her ideal body weight. Growth and weight gain are continuously monitored (sometimes weekly in infants). If a child is obese, the calories are calculated to gradually—over several months—bring him toward his ideal weight. If the child is gaining weight in excess of growth, calories are reduced. **Weight gain is due to excess *calories* ingested, not to excess *fat* ingestion.** If a child is not growing adequately, we may adjust the ratio or add more protein to the diet.

LIPIDS: Society has been taught and retaught that a high-fat diet will elevate cholesterol and triglycerides and lead to strokes and heart attacks. We have been taught to eat low-fat or nonfat foods. **What are the effects of a 90 percent fat diet on cholesterol and on lipids?** We have been carefully monitoring the lipids of all our children while they are on the diet. An abstract of some of these data are shown in Figure 11-5.

As can be seen, when the children are switched from a normal diet to a 90 percent fat diet, both the cholesterol and the triglycerides are elevated. Cholesterol seems to go from a high-normal level in the 160 to 220 range. Such a level, if maintained for a lifetime, is thought to increase the risk of heart disease and stroke.

However, the ketogenic diet is *not* maintained for a lifetime. In general, it is continued for three years or more if it is effective in controlling the seizures. Half of the children discontinue the diet before one year because it is too difficult or too ineffective. In such cases the children return to a normal lower fat diet and the lipids should return to their pre-diet state. If the child is to continue on the ketogenic diet for many years, consideration should be given to the relative risks of the higher lipids compared with the risks of the medications and seizures.

We have seen several children whose lipids go very high—cholesterol of more than 800 mg/dl and triglycerides over 1000 mg/dl. Even with these levels, our lipid experts tell us that the diet need not be discontinued—if it is beneficial. We are told that these levels are unlikely to cause

FIGURE 11-5
Lipid profile and the ketogenic diet.

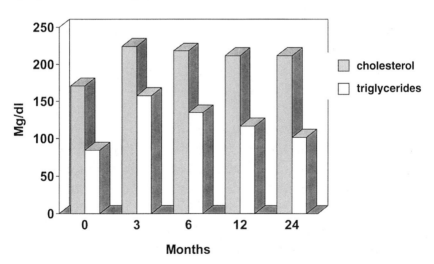

stroke or heart disease unless they are maintained for years. The acute concern of such levels is pancreatitis (inflammation of the pancreas). Reducing the diet ratio from 4:1 to 3.5:1 in these children has had a dramatic effect on lowering the lipids to reasonable levels. Again, parents and physicians must weigh risks and benefits of alternative courses of action.

BETA-HYDROXYBUTYRIC ACID (BOHB): Beta-hydroxybutyric acid and acetone are the two important ketone bodies left when fats are incompletely "burned" by the body in the absence of sufficient ketones. Acetone is usually expelled in the breath and gives the sweet smell to the breath that is present in children who are in good ketosis. On the other hand, BOHB is largely metabolized in the body and excreted in the urine, giving the positive ketostick test. It is believed that it is the BOHB that in some way has anticonvulsant properties.

The ketogenic diet has been based on modifying the child's calories and diet ratio so that the urine tests 3+ to 4+ (80–160 mml) on the ketosticks. This is a crude test, but direct measurement of the ketones in the blood has until now been expensive and required a needle stick. However, we have known for decades that while it was necessary to have 3–4+ ketones in the urine, that level was not necessarily sufficient for good seizure control. We have known that if a child who had 3–4+ urinary ketones was still having seizures, decreasing the calories or raising the ratio might improve control. We also knew that increasing the child's fluid intake might dilute the urine and lower the value on the test strip.

We believe that we are on the verge of a major change in how we assess ketosis and how we adjust the diet to obtain optimal ketosis. It is possible that we can obtain even better seizure control in the future by monitoring serum ketone bodies by finger prick.

New approaches to measuring beta-hydroxybutyric acid on finger-stick blood are in the process of development. In the near future, children on the ketogenic diet will likely have their BOHB monitored at home by their parents, much as blood sugar is now monitored in those with diabetes. It is hoped, but as of this writing unproven, that this will lead to even more effective seizure control with the diet.

CARNITINE: We have found no evidence that the ketogenic diet causes carnitine deficiency. Since it is difficult to measure carnitine deficiency, if a child seems to become weak or frail, begins to have frequent illnesses, or just is not doing well, then we may give the child supplemental carnitine (100 mg/kg.) **for one month.** If indeed there was carnitine deficiency, then the child should show a dramatic improvement in symptoms, and we would continue the supplement. We are unaware of this occurring in our patients. However, we have heard of several children whose carnitine deficiency was unmasked by the diet and who have shown dramatic improvement with additional carnitine supplementation.

HOW DOES THE DIET WORK

The BIG question—how does the diet work—remains to be answered. But now that it has been reestablished that the diet works, there is ongoing laboratory and animal research to identify the mechanisms by which it might be effective in controlling seizures of different types, or different causes, and in children of different ages. Understanding the mechanisms of the anticonvulsant action of the ketogenic diet might also provide new insights into some of the basic mechanisms underlying the epilepsies and lead to even better and less difficult approaches to its treatment.

Perhaps we can wish that such insights will be part of the next edition of this book.

CHAPTER TWELVE

CONCLUSION

If this book causes one child to avoid having a seizure or to decrease the fog that may accompany high doses of medication, we will have achieved one of our goals. Having witnessed the success of the ketogenic diet at the Pediatric Epilepsy Center at Johns Hopkins, we know how effective the ketogenic diet can be. If we can make it available to increasing numbers of children at medical centers across the country and beyond, through improved documentation and the ease of an improved computer program, another goal will have been realized.

The use of the ketogenic diet is becoming more widespread as prejudice and fears among professionals and parents are dispelled: prejudice among physicians against "alternative medicine" that does not come in a neat antiseptic package; skepticism among parents about whether the benefits of the diet will be worth the loss of food freedom; anxiety among dietitians about the subtleties of the diet calculation. If this book, the computer program, and the videos help to overcome these fears and prejudices, a third goal will have been surpassed.

This book has been written primarily about the diet as administered to young children. Its success in adolescents remains to be fully tested, but motivation and compliance, rather than the diet itself, appear to be the major impediments. The use and effectiveness of the diet in adults has been studied even less. Perhaps by the next edition of this book enough data will have been collected to add a chapter on these age groups.

The overwhelming enthusiasm of parents who have tried the diet, independent of their own success, has motivated many medical centers to establish ketogenic diet programs of their own. We hope that each center, each parent, and each child experiences success.

But our ultimate goal is more far-reaching. Within the ketogenic diet may lie an as yet undiscovered metabolic key to the puzzle of why seizures and epilepsy occur in the first place and how they can be treated more effectively.

As clinical and laboratory investigation turn their attention to the diet and if researchers can decipher how the ketogenic diet brings seizures to an end, we can possibly discover a medication that will block seizures. Ideally this future medication will have no side effects and be as effective as the diet but without its rigor and sacrifice. Since this book was first written, we have learned much about the ketogenic diet. We can hope that the ketogenic diet will be the start of a new era in the understanding and treatment of seizures and epilepsy.

SECTION VI

APPENDIXES

MEDICATIONS

1. GENERAL RULES

- Find one pharmacist who is willing to become knowledgeable about the ketogenic diet and monitor all medications and pharmaceutical products.

- Medications should be taken only in the form prescribed, as carbohydrate and sugar concentrations vary from liquids to tablets to caplets even if made by the same manufacturer.

- Ideally, your physician will order all medications from a compounding pharmacy in sugar-free or carbohydrate-free form. Locate a compounding pharmacy in your area if possible.

- In the event of emergency room treatment or hospital admission, intravenous solutions should be normal saline, not glucose or lactated ringers. Medications in a hospital setting should be given rectally or intravenously whenever possible as these forms usually have lower carbohydrate levels.

- In the event of a life-threatening emergency, the child's immediate need for stabilization comes first. All medical personnel should be advised about the diet and advised that seizure activity may increase with glucose administration.

2. SOURCES OF INFORMATION

Abbott Laboratories	1-800-633-9110
Bristol-Meyers Squibb	1-800-321-1335
Carter-Wallace	1-609-655-6000
Eli Lilly Laboratories	1-800-545-5979
Glaxo Wellcome	1-800-722-9292
MeadJohnson Nutritionals	1-812-429-5000
McNeil Consumer Health Care	1-215-273-7000
Novartis	1-888-644-8585
Parke-Davis	1-800-223-0432
Procter & Gamble	1-800-358-8707
Roche Laboratories	1-800-526-6367
Ross Products Division	1-614-624-7677
Roxane Laboratories	1-800-848-0120
SmithKline Beecham	1-800-233-2426
Pharmacia & Upjohn	1-616-329-8244
Scot-Tussin Pharmacal Co.	1-800-638-7268
Shine Pharmaceuticals	1-800-356-5790
Teva Pharmaceuticals USA	1-201-703-0400
Warner-Chilcott Laboratories	1-800-424-5202
Wyeth-Ayerst Laboratories	1-800-544-9871

3. MEDICATIONS COMMONLY USED BY CHILDREN ON THE KETOGENIC DIET

The following is not intended to be a comprehensive list. There may be other medications available in each category that contain no sugar, starch, or carbohydrates, and as formulations change, some of the medications listed here may be disallowed in the future. It is important to pay close attention to labeling and to contact the manufacturer in case of doubt.

All medications on these lists contain minimal carbohydrate and may be used with the diet unless otherwise indicated. If a medication contains less than one gram of carbohydrate per dose, it need not be calculated into the diet.

Most liquid preparations contain large amounts of sugar or sugar substitutes. Check with manufacturer. Tablets may be a good alternative. Crushing tablets may destroy the medication in some cases, however, so check with a pharmacist if you wish to crush tablets. Children can weather most colds without the use of over-the-counter medications.

Antiepileptic Medications

Carbatrol (Shire Richwood)	200 mg tab — 20 mg lactose
	300 mg tab — 30 mg lactose
	Remove from shell and use as sprinkles.
	Shell contains 60–90 mg sugar
Depakote (Abbott)	125 mg sprinkles — no carbohydrate
	(minute amounts of magnesium
	stearate in the gel capsule)
Depakote (Abbott)	125 mg tab — 25 mg starch
	250 mg tab — 50 mg starch
	500 mg tab — 100 mg starch
Dilantin (Parke-Davis)	30 mg capsule — 72 mg sucrose,
	74 mg lactose
	100 mg capsule — 58 mg sucrose,
	74 mg lactose
	Avoid use of Infatabs or liquid preparation
Felbamate (Wallace)	400 mg tab — 87 mg starch,
	40 mg lactose
	600 mg tab — 130 mg starch,
	60 mg lactose
	Suspension — 1500 mg/5 ml sorbitol.
	Do not use.

Gapapentin (Parke-Davis)	100 mg cap — 14.25 mg lactose, 10 mg starch
	300 mg cap — 42.75 mg lactose, 30 mg starch
	400 mg cap — 57 mg lactose, 40 mg starch
Mysoline (Wyeth-Ayerst)	50 mg tab — 27.7 mg lactose, 4.4 mg starch
	250 mg tab — 22.4 mg lactose, 12 mg starch
	Suspension — .75 mg/ml saccharine sodium (this is the only sweetener)
Tegretol (Novartis)	200 mg tab — 51.5 mg starch
	Avoid use of the 100 mg chewable or liquid preparation.
Tegretol X-R (Novartis)	100 mg tab — 28 mg dextrate
	200 mg tab — 56 mg dextrate
Zarontin (Parke-Davis)	250 mg cap — 51.1 mg sorbitol
	Suspension — 625mg/5cc sorbitol — Do not use
Phenobarbital (Danbury)	30 mg tabs — 48 mg lactose, 18 mg starch

Remember: Formulations may change
without notification from the manufacturer!

Antibiotics

Antibiotics commonly used by children on the ketogenic diet:

- Septra tablets (Glaxo Wellcome). Single or double strength
- Ampicillin (Squibb). 250 and 500 mg. capsules
- Augmentin (SmithKline Beecham). 250 mg. and 500 mg. white-coated tablets or oral suspension powder (not chewable tablets or pre-mixed suspension)
- Ceclor (Lilly). 250 mg. capsule (not suspension)
- Ceftin (Glaxo). 125 mg., 250 mg., and 500 mg tablets
- Erythromycin (Abbott). 250 mg. and 500 mg. film-coated tablets or time-release capsule

Cough and Cold Preparations

Cold and cough remedies commonly used by children on the ketogenic diet:

- Benadryl Decongestant/Allergy Tablets (Parke-Davis)
- Benadryl Allergy/Sinus/Headache Tablets
- Benadryl Cold/Flu Tablets
  *Benadryl Allergy contains lactose;
  Dye-Free Allergy contains sorbitol. Do not use.*
- Comtrex Multi-Symptom Cold & Flu Tablets (Bristol Myers Squibb)
- Diabetic Tussin DM (Hi-Tech Pharmaceutical Co., Inc.). Cough suppressant/expectorant.
- Drixoral Cold & Flu Tablets — 12 Hour Formula (Schering Plough). *Drixoral Cold & Allergy formula contains lactose and sugar. Do not use.*
- Scot-Tussin DM
- Tylenol Cold Gelcaps (McNeil)
- Tylenol PM Caplets

Laxatives and Stool Softeners

Constipation is a chronic problem for many children on the ketogenic diet. Laxatives, enemas, and to a lesser extent suppositories can cause dependency when used on a regular basis. Whenever possible, try to rely on less invasive measures such as stool softeners and natural bulk fiber. In order for any of these remedies to work effectively, sufficient fluid intake must be maintained. Be sure your child is receiving up to his full fluid restriction and offer fluids at the time of medication administration. In particularly severe cases of constipation, talk to your doctor or dietitian about increasing fluid allowances.

- Colace capsules or 1% Solution (Apothecon).
  Stool softener. *Do not use syrup.*

- Dulcolax suppositories (CIBA Consumer)

- Fleet enema (Fleet). Use only small amount and
  only occasionally. Can cause dependence.

- Glycerin suppositories

- MCT oil (see p. 32)

- Mineral oil. Laxative that is not absorbed by the body,
  but may carry essential body nutrients with it during
  elimination. May be used occasionally.

- Pepto-Bismol Original or Maximum Strength Liquid.
  Anti-diarrheal. *Do not use caplets or chewable tablets.*

- Peri-Colace Capsules (Apothecon). Stool softener and
  laxative. Use only after you have tried regular Colace first.

- Phillips' Milk of Magnesia (original flavor only).

Pain Relievers

- Aleve Tablets.
- Motrin IB Capsules (Upjohn)
- Nuprin Coated Tablets (Bristol Myers Squibb)
- Tempra (Bristol-Meyers Squibb). Infant drops
  Do not use tablets or pediatric elixirs.
- Tylenol (McNeil). Original flavor infant drops, suppositories, or regular/extra-strength tablets. *Do not use pediatric elixirs.*

Vitamin and Mineral Supplements

Liquid supplements are generally recommended for children under a year to three years of age. For older children, give one and a half to two times the dose or give supplements in tablet form. Iron preparations must be given mixed with food as direct contact with teeth can cause black spots.

- Calcium carbonate (Rugby or Giant). 600–650 mg. tablets.
- Carnitor 330 mg. capsules
  Liquid contains sugar. Do not use
- Fields of Nature makes many individual vitamin supplements for children with specific deficiencies.
- Lactaid Drops (McNeil Consumer Products).
  Lactaid Caplets contain mannitol. Do not use.
- One-A-Day Essential Multi-Vitamin
  (tablet form for older children)
- One-A-Day Maximum Multi-Vitamin
- Poly-Vi-Sol Drops with iron.
  Do not give Poly-Vi-Sol in tablet form.
- Unicap M (Multi-Vitamin in tablet form)
- Vi-Daylin Drops with iron.
  Do not give in tablet form.

Toothpastes and Mouthwashes

- Arm & Hammer Dental Care toothpaste
- Listermint mouthwash (Warner-Lambert)
- Plax Dental Rinse — original or mint
  (Consumer Health Care Group)
- Scope — peppermint/mint/baking soda (Proctor & Gamble)
- Tom's of Maine toothpaste
- Ultra Brite toothpaste (Colgate-Palmolive)

MCT Oil

MCT oil can be obtained from MeadJohnson Nutritionals at a cost of approximately $80 per quart.

It can also be obtained from K.C. Enterprises, a distributor for the Ultimate Nutrition Company. The product is called MCT Gold. It may be ordered at 1-800-305-0951. The cost is $17.50/liter plus $5.00 shipping charge.

JOHNS HOPKINS
HOSPITAL NURSING
CRITICAL PATHWAYS

DEPARTMENT OF PEDIATRICS
KETOGENIC DIET
CRITICAL PATHWAY

Primary Nurse: _____
Case Manager: _____
Attending: _____
Date Initiated: _____
Date discussed with patient/family: _____

for addressograph plate

NAME: _____
DATE: _____

	Clinic	Hospital Day 1	Hospital Day 2	Hospital Day 3	Hospital Day 4	Hospital Day 5		
MONITORING/ ASSESSMENT		Neuro checks q 6° **Be alert to S&S of** hypoglycemia!! OR Medication toxicity Monitor seizure activity # of seizures described on flowsheet Nutrition assessment						
TREATMENTS								

NAME: _____ DATE: _____

	Clinic	Hospital Day 1	Hospital Day 2	Hospital Day 3	Hospital Day 4	Hospital Day 5	
MEDICATIONS	Home routine drugs transition to standard sugar-free antiepileptic drugs *Total meds must have ▼ .1 gm carbohydrate q day		1) Caltrate 600 or Calcimix 2) Unicap M or Poly-Vi-Sol with iron		Glycerin suppository if no BM since admission		
ACTIVITY	Ad lib as tolerated	Ad lib Child Life to playroom	Child Life Assessment				
DIET	NPO after evening meal except clear diet caffeine-free liquids: water, diet Shasta, weak caffeine-free tea	NPO until ▲ 48 hrs and 4 (+) ketones in urine established (¾ maintenance) 60–70cc kg fluid Orange juice 30cc for BS ▼ 40 if symptoms of hypoglycemia	⅓ total diet × 3 meals (eggnog formula) as per nutrition consult sheet *Each change in diet must have order written specifying; *Calories, gms CHO, protein, +fat and ratio (Total per Meal)*	⅓ total diet × 3 meals (eggnog formula)	Full regular ketogenic diet until discharge (7th meal)	Discharge with travel eggnog (2 meals)	
TESTS	AM out-patient EEG if not done in past 6 months	Heme 8, Urinalysis M7, M12 AED levels Lipid profile- (hand carried to lipid lab- m6-110)					

NAME: _____   DATE: _____

TESTS (cont'd)	✓ Ketones q void Glucose ✓ q6• until 2/3 diet established q2• if ▼40					
CONSULTS	Nutrition consult daily — dietitian Social work consult					
PATIENT TEACHING	Family version of path shared with patient and family Meeting with dietician — 1 p.m. Out-patient clinic appointment History and theory of keto diet Fats, carbohydrates, and proteins Ketogenic vs. non-ketogenic potential Components of the diet (i.e., ratio, calories, fluid, etc.)	Parents have access to ketogenic diet book and parent teaching tape ☐ Yes ☐ No Parents know how to check urine for ketones ☐ Yes ☐ No Review meal plans and food exchanges Parents assist with planning meals to be eaten during the hospital stay	Meal preparation instruction Review scale and measuring technique Discussion of commercial products that can and cannot be used on diet Label reading: How to find hidden sugars Medication review Continue to discuss meal planning options	Review previous material Answer questions Discuss complications that may occur at home and remedies: nausea/hunger constipation refusal to eat illness, etc. low ketosis lethargy	Role playing with older children What to say when offered food How to tell others about the special diet Importance of not cheating, even once	

NAME: _____   DATE: _____

	Clinic	Hospital Day 1	Hospital Day 2	Hospital Day 3	Hospital Day 4	Hospital Day 5		
DISCHARGE PLANNING	Teaching Interactive met □Yes □No	Parents given meal plans □Yes □No	Parents given meal plans □Yes □No Parents must have scale and graduated cylinder for teaching. □Yes □No Prescriptions for AEDs, calcium and vitamin supply, urine dip sticks □Yes □No					
EVALUATION OF OUTCOMES		Seizure □Yes □No 4 + Ketones □Yes □No NPO □Yes □No	Seizure □Yes □No 4 + Ketones □Yes □No 1/3 diet □Yes □No	Seizure □Yes □No 4 + Ketones □Yes □No 1/3 diet □Yes □No	Seizure □Yes □No 4 + Ketones □Yes □No 2/3 diet (eggnog) □Yes □No	Seizure □Yes □No 4 + Ketones □Yes □No Full ketogenic diet □Yes □No		

NAME: _____   DATE: _____

EVALUATION OF OUTCOMES (cont'd)

Title		Signature						
Night	P / A	Electrolytes WNL □Yes □No	Child Life Assessment □Yes □No	²/₃ diet □Yes □No	Full diet □Yes □No	P / A	P / A	P / A
Day	P / A	Family version of path shared □Yes □No	Social Work Assessment □Yes □No	Follow-up scheduled □Yes □No		P / A	P / A	P / A
Evening	P / A		Parents demonstrate how to check urine for ketones □Yes □No	Parents demonstrate ability to accurately weigh foods using a gram scale □Yes □No	Parents can write a meal plan with specific foods and weights for several complete days □Yes □No	P / A	P / A	P / A
			Parents can demonstrate correct use of food exchanges in a sample meal plan □Yes □No	Parents can read a product label and determine whether it is appropriate for the keto diet □Yes □No	Parents can describe possible complications of the diet and their remedies □Yes □No			
			Parents can calculate total fluid allotment for a given day □Yes □No	Parents have Rx for calcium, anti-epileptic drugs, vitamin supply and urine dip sticks □Yes □No				

APPENDIX C

SELECTED

REFERENCES

GENERAL INFORMATION ON EPILEPSY

Freeman JM, Vining EPG, and Pillas DJ, *Seizures and Epilepsy: A Guide for Parents.* Johns Hopkins University Press, Baltimore. 1990, 1996.

RECENT REFERENCES ON THE EFFECTIVENESS AND ACCEPTABILITY OF THE KETOGENIC DIET

Blue Cross–Blue Shield Technology Assessment Program Ketogenic Diet for the Treatment of Children with Refractory Epilepsy. Tec Vol. 15, No. 20, pp. 1–27, October 1998.

Casey JC, Vining EPG, Freeman JM, et al. The implementation and maintenance of the ketogenic diet in children. *J Neurosci Nurs* 1999; 31:294–302.

Freeman JM, Vining EPG. Seizures rapidly decrease after fasting: preliminary studies of the ketogenic diet. *Arch Pediatr Adolesc* 1999; 153; 946–949.

Freeman JM, Vining EPG, Pillas DJ, Pyzik PL, Casey JC, Kelly MT. The efficacy of the ketogenic diet—1998: a prospective evaluation of intervention in 150 children. *Pediatrics* 1998; 102: 1358–1363.

Furth S, Fivush B, Freeman JM, Vining EPG. Kidney stones and the ketogenic diet: studies in prevention and treatment. *Pediatr Nephrol* 2000, in press

Gilbert DL, Pyzik PL, Vining EPG, Freeman JM. Medication cost reduction in children on the ketogenic diet: data from a prospective study of 150 children over one year. *J Child Neurol* 1999; 14:469–471.

LeFever G, Aronson N. Ketogenic diet for the treatment of refractory epilepsy in children: a systematic review of efficacy. *Pediatrics* 2000; 105(4) (Abstract). URL: http://www.pediatrics.org/cgi/content/full/4/e46.

Schwartzkroin PA. Mechanisms underlying the anti-epileptic efficacy of the ketogenic diet. *Epilepsy Res* 1999; 37:171–180.

Stafstrom CE. Animal models of the ketogenic diet: what have we learned, what can we learn? *Epilepsy Res* 1999; 37: 241–259.

Swink TD, Vining EPG, Freeman JM, The ketogenic diet 1996, *Adv Pediatr* 1997; 44: 297–329.

Vining EPG, Freeman JM, for the Ketogenic Diet Study Group. A multicenter study of the efficacy of the ketogenic diet. *Arch Neurol* 1998; 55:1433–1437.

OTHER BOOKS OF INTEREST

Keith, Haddow M. *Convulsive Disorders in Children: With Reference to Treatment with the Ketogenic Diet.* Little, Brown and Company, Boston. 1963, Chapters 12 & 13.

Lennox, William G. *Epilepsy and Related Disorders.* Little, Brown and Company, Boston. 1960. Vol 2:734–739, 824–832.

Livingston, S. *Living with Epileptic Seizures.* Charles C. Thomas, Springfield, Ill. 1963:143–163.

Livingston, Samuel. *The Diagnosis and Treatment of Convulsive Disorders in Children.* Charles C. Thomas, Springfield, Ill. 1954:213–236.

THE MEDIUM-CHAIN TRIGLYCERIDE (MCT) DIET

Huttenlocher PR, Wilbourn AJ, Signore JM. Medium-chain triglycerides as a therapy for intractable epilepsy. *Neurology* 1971;21:1097–1103.

Sills MA, Forsyth WI, Haidukwych D. The medium-chain triglyceride diet and intractable epilepsy. *Arch Disease in Childhood* 1986:1169–1172.

Trauner, DA. Medium-chain triglyceride (MCT) diet in intractable seizure disorders. *Neurology* 1985:237–238.

OTHER ARTICLES OF INTEREST

De Vivo DC, Pagliara AS, Prensky AL. Ketotic hypoglycemia and the ketogenic diet. *Neurology* 1973;23:640–649.

Dodson WE, Prensky AL, De Vivo DC, Goldring S, Dodge PR. Management of seizure disorders: selected aspects. Part II. *J Pediatr* 1976;89:695–703.

Herzberg GZ, Fivush BA, Kinsman SL, Gearhart JP. Urolithiasis associated with the ketogenic diet. *J Pediatr* 1990;117:743–745.

Livingston S, Pauli S, Pruce I. Ketogenic diet in the treatment of childhood epilepsy. *Dev Med Child Neurol* 1977;19:833–834.

Millichap JG, Jones JD, Rudis BP. Mechanism of anticonvulsant action of ketogenic diet. *Am J Dis Child* 1964;107:593–603.

Withrow CD. Antiepileptic drugs. The ketogenic diet: mechanism of anticonvulsant action. In: Glaser GH, Penry JK, Woodbury DM, eds. *Antiepileptic Drugs: Mechanisms of Action.* New York: Raven Press, 1980:635–642.

SELECTED EXPERIMENTAL STUDIES OF THE DIET IN ANIMALS

Appleton DB, De Vivo DC. An animal model for the ketogenic diet. Electroconvulsive threshold and biochemical alterations consequent upon high-fat diet. *Epilepsia* 1974;15:211–227.

De Vivo DC, Malas KL, Leckie MP. Starvation and seizures. Observations on the electroconvulsive threshold and cerebral metabolism of the starved adult rat. *Arch Neurol* 1975;32:755–760.

Mahoney AW, Hendricks DG, Bernhard N, Sisson DV. Fasting and ketogenic diet effects on audiogenic seizure susceptibility in magnesium deficient rats. *Pharmacol Biochem Behav* 1983;18:683–687.

FOOD

DATABASE

The Epilepsy Diet Treatment Food List

Category	Code	Description	Grams	Protein	Fat	Carb	Kcal
BABY	BAPAP	Gerber Apple/Apricot	100	0.22	0.22	11.63	49
	BAPPA	Gerber Apple/Pineapple	100	0.08	0.08	10.08	41
	BAPPL	Strained Apples	100	0.16	0.16	10.94	46
	BAPRA	Gerber Apple/Raspberry	100	0.22	0.15	15.17	63
	BBATA	Gerber Banana Tapioca	100	0.37	0.07	15.26	63
	BBEEF	Strained Beef	100	13.64	5.35	0.00	103
	BBEET	Strained Beets	100	1.33	0.08	7.66	37
	BCARR	Strained Carrots	100	0.78	0.16	6.02	29
	BCHIC	Strained Chicken	100	13.74	7.88	0.10	126
	BGRBE	Strained Green Beans	100	1.33	0.08	5.94	30
	BLAMB	Strained Lamb	100	14.04	4.75	0.10	99
	BMIXV	Strained Mixed Vegetables	100	1.25	0.47	7.97	41
	BPEAC	Strained Peaches	100	0.52	0.15	18.89	79
	BPEAR	Strained Pears	100	0.31	0.16	10.86	46
	BPEAS	Strained Peas	100	3.52	0.31	8.13	49
	BPEPA	Strained Pear/Pineapple	100	0.31	0.08	10.86	45
	BSQUA	Strained Squash	100	0.86	0.16	5.63	27
	BTURK	Strained Turkey	100	15.35	7.07	0.00	125
	BAPBL	Gerber Apple/Blueberry	100	0.22	0.22	16.30	68
DAIRY	CHAM	American Cheese, Kraft/Land O Lake	100	19.05	23.81	9.52	329
	CHCH	Cheddar Cheese, Kraft/Land O Lake	100	21.43	32.14	3.57	389
	CHCO	Cottage Cheese, 2% Lowfat	100	13.16	2.19	2.63	83
	CHCR	Cream Cheese, Philadelphia Brand	100	6.67	33.33	3.33	340
	CHMON	Monterey Cheese	100	24.64	30.71	0.71	378

Category	Code	Description	Grams	Protein	Fat	Carb	Kcal
DAIRY (cont'd)	CHMOZ	Mozzarella Cheese, Whole Milk	100	21.43	25.00	3.57	325
	CHPAR	Parmesan, Grated	100	42.00	30.00	4.00	454
	CHSW	Swiss Cheese	100	24.50	24.85	2.10	332
	CHWZ	Cheez Whiz, Kraft	100	16.43	20.36	6.43	275
	CREA1	Cream, 36%	100	2.00	36.00	3.00	344
	CREA2	Cream 30%	100	2.00	30.67	2.67	295
	EGG	Egg, Fresh	100	12.00	9.00	1.20	134
	SOUR	Sour Cream	100	3.33	16.67	6.67	190
	YOGUR	Yogurt, Plain Lowfat	100	5.24	1.54	7.05	63
	CHMOZ2	Mozzarella Cheese, Part Skim	100	28.57	17.86	3.57	289
	CHCO2	Cottage Cheese 4% Lowfat	100	13.16	4.39	3.51	106
	CHRC	Ricotta Cheese, Whole Milk	100	9.68	12.90	6.45	181
	CHRC2	Ricotta Cheese, Part Skim	100	10.34	7.76	6.90	139
	WHMK	Whole Milk (ML)	100	3.39	3.39	5.02	64
FATS	BUTT	Butter	100	0.67	81.33	0.00	735
	MARG	Margarine, Stick Corn	100	0.00	76.00	0.00	684
	MAYO	Mayonnaise, Hellman	100	1.43	80.00	0.70	729
	OILC	Corn Oil	100	0.00	97.14	0.00	874
	OILO	Olive Oil	100	0.00	96.43	0.00	868
	OILP	Puritan Oil	100	0.00	100.00	0.00	900
	OILM	MCT Oil	100	0.00	92.67	0.00	834
FISH	FLOU	Flounder, Baked	100	24.12	1.53	0.00	110
	HADD	Haddock, Baked	100	24.30	0.95	0.00	106
	LOBST	Lobster, Raw	100	18.82	0.94	0.47	86
	REDS	Red Snapper, Raw	100	26.35	1.76	0.00	121

Category	Code	Description	Grams	Protein	Fat	Carb	Kcal
FISH	SALM	Salmon, Raw	100	20.00	3.41	0.00	111
(cont'd)	SCAL	Scallops, Raw	100	16.82	0.71	2.35	83
	SHRIM	Shrimp, Raw	100	20.35	1.76	0.94	101
	SWORD	Swordfish, Baked	100	25.41	5.18	0.00	148
	TROUT	Rainbow Trout	100	26.35	4.35	0.00	145
	TUNA1	Tuna Lt Chnk StarKist/Oil	100	22.41	22.41	0.00	291
	TUNA2	Tuna Lt Chnk StarKist/Water	100	23.21	0.89	0.00	101
	TUNA3	Tuna All White StarKist/Water	100	21.43	8.93	0.00	166
	TUNA4	Tuna, Fresh	100	29.88	6.24	0.00	175
FRUIT	APPLE	Apple	100	0.21	0.36	14.84	63
	APPLS	Applesauce, Unsweetened	100	0.16	0.08	11.31	47
	APRI	Apricot	100	1.42	0.38	11.13	54
	BANAN	Banana	100	1.05	0.53	23.42	103
	BLUE	Blueberries	100	0.69	0.41	14.14	63
	CANT	Cantaloupe	100	0.88	0.25	8.38	39
	CHERR	Cherries	100	1.18	1.03	16.62	80
	FRCOC	Fruit Cocktail Canned/Water	100	0.41	0.08	8.52	36
	GRAFR	Grapefruit, Pink	100	0.57	0.08	7.72	34
	GRAPG	Green Grapes	100	0.65	0.33	17.17	74
	GRAPP	Purple Grapes	100	0.69	0.56	17.75	79
	HONML	Honeydew Melon	100	0.80	0.30	7.70	37
	JAPP	Apple Juice	100	0.10	0.10	11.70	48
	JORAN	Orange Juice	100	0.70	0.20	10.40	46
	LEMON	Lemon	100	1.03	0.34	9.31	44
	LEMRI	Lemon Rind	100	1.67	0.00	16.67	73
	MANGO	Mango	100	0.53	0.29	17.00	73

Category	Code	Description	Grams	Protein	Fat	Carb	Kcal
FRUIT (cont'd)	NECT	Nectarine	100	0.96	0.44	11.76	55
	ORANG	Orange, Navel	100	1.00	0.07	11.64	51
	PEACH	Peach	100	0.69	0.11	11.15	48
	PEAR	Pear	100	0.42	0.42	15.12	66
	PINEA	Pineapple	100	0.39	0.45	12.39	55
	PLUM	Plum	100	0.76	0.61	13.03	61
	PUMPK	Pumpkin, Canned	100	1.07	0.25	8.11	39
	RASP	Raspberries	100	0.89	0.57	11.54	55
	STRAW	Strawberries	100	0.60	0.40	7.05	34
	TANG	Tangerine	100	0.60	0.24	11.19	49
	WATML	Watermelon	100	0.63	0.44	7.19	35
GENERIC	GMFP	Generic Meat, Fish, Poultry	100	23.30	16.70	0.00	243
	GFRU	Generic 10% Fruit Exchange	100	1.00	0.00	10.00	44
	GVEG	Generic Group B Vegetable Exchange	100	2.00	0.00	7.00	36
	GPBUT	Generic Peanut Butter Exchange	100	26.00	48.00	22.00	624
	GFAT	Generic Butter, Margarine, Mayo	100	0.00	74.00	0.00	666
	GSTMT	Generic Strained Meats	100	13.33	6.67	0.00	113
MEAT	BACO	Bacon, Oscar Mayer	100	33.33	41.67	0.00	508
	BEEF1	Eye Round Beef	100	29.00	6.50	0.00	175
	BEEF2	Lean Ground Beef Medium	100	24.20	19.10	0.00	269
	BOLO1	Beef Bologna, Oscar Mayer	100	10.71	28.57	3.57	314
	BOLO2	Beef Bologna, Hebrew National	100	10.71	10.71	2.86	151
	CANBAC	Canadian Bacon, Oscar Mayer	100	19.58	4.17	0.42	118
	CORBF	Corned Beef, Oscar Mayer	100	20.00	1.76	0.59	98
	HAM	Cured Ham, Center Slice	100	20.20	12.90	0.10	197

Category	Code	Description	Grams	Protein	Fat	Carb	Kcal
MEAT (cont'd)	HOTD1	Beef Frank, Hebrew National	100	12.50	29.17	2.08	321
	HOTD2	Beef Frank Oscar Mayer	100	11.11	28.89	2.22	313
	LAMB	Leg of Lamb, Lean	100	28.71	7.06	0.00	178
	LEAN	Lean and Tasty	100	23.30	35.80	0.80	419
	PORK	Pork Chop, Lean Broiled	100	32.00	10.50	0.00	223
	SAUS1	Oscar Mayer Pork, Beef Link	100	13.30	27.80	2.20	312
	SAUS2	Sausage, Bob Evans	100	13.57	30.71	2.50	341
	SAUS3	Sausage, Hillshire Farm	100	12.28	29.82	3.51	332
	VEAL	Veal Cutlet	100	27.06	11.06	0.00	208
MISC	CHOC1	Baking Chocolate, Bakers	100	11.07	52.14	30.00	634
	CHOC2	Baking Chocolate, Hershey's	100	14.29	56.43	23.93	661
	COCOA	Hershey's Cocoa	100	27.30	12.80	45.70	407
	JELLO	Jello Sugar Free Gelatin	100	1.16	0.00	0.17	5
	MUST1	Mustard Yellow	100	4.00	4.00	6.00	76
	OLIV1	Olives, Green	100	1.09	10.65	1.09	105
	OLIV2	Olives, Black	100	1.67	28.75	7.08	294
	SOY	Soy Sauce	100	10.52	0.17	5.52	66
	TARTA	Tartar Sauce, Kraft	100	0.00	64.29	0.00	579
	VINEG	Vinegar, Distilled	100	0.00	0.00	5.33	21
NUTS	ALMON	Almonds, Dry Roasted	100	16.43	52.50	24.64	637
	BRAZ	Brazil Nuts	100	14.64	67.14	12.86	714
	CASH	Cashews, Dry Roasted	100	15.71	47.14	34.29	624
	MACAD	Macadamia Nuts	100	8.57	75.71	8.93	751
	PEAN1	Peanuts, Dry Roasted	100	23.57	49.64	21.43	627
	PEAN2	Peanuts, Oil Roasted	100	29.64	48.57	16.07	620

Category	Code	Description	Grams	Protein	Fat	Carb	Kcal
NUTS (cont'd)	PECAN	Pecans	100	8.21	65.71	22.50	714
	PETE	Peter Pan Pan Chunky Peanut Butter	100	25.00	50.00	22.00	638
	PIST	Pistachio Nuts	100	15.00	53.57	27.86	654
	SKIP	Skippy Creamy Peanut Butter	100	28.13	53.13	15.60	653
	SUNF	Sunflower Seeds	100	23.21	50.36	18.93	622
	WALN	Walnuts, Black, Dried	100	24.64	57.50	12.14	665
POULTRY	CHIC	Chicken Breast—No Skin (Cooked)	100	31.05	3.60	0.00	157
	TURK	Turkey Breast	100	29.90	3.20	0.00	148
SOUP	BOUL1	Wylers Inst Boull—Chicken/Beef	100	0.00	0.00	28.57	114
	BROTH1	Swanson Canned—Chicken (ML)	100	0.83	0.83	0.42	12
	BROTH2	Swanson Canned—Beef (ML)	100	0.83	0.42	0.42	9
	BROTH3	Swanson Canned—Vegetable (ML)	100	0.00	10.42	1.25	9
TUBE	TMICR	Microlipid (ML)	100	0.00	50.00	0.00	450
	TPLOY	Polycose Powder	100	0.00	0.00	94.00	376
	TRCFC	RCF Concentration (ML)	100	4.00	7.20	0.00	81
VEGETABLE	ASPAR	Asparagus—C (Grp A)	100	2.56	0.33	4.44	31
	BEAN1	Green Beans	100	1.94	0.32	7.90	42
	BEET	Beets—C (Grp B)	100	1.06	0.00	6.71	31
	BROC	Broccoli—C (Grp B)	100	2.95	0.25	5.50	36
	BRUS	Brussels Sprouts	100	2.56	0.51	8.31	48
	CABB1	Cabbage, Green—R	100	1.14	0.29	5.43	29
	CABB2	Cabbage, Green—C	100	0.93	0.13	4.80	24
	CARR	Carrots—R or C (Grp B)	100	1.15	0.13	10.50	48

Category	Code	Description	Grams	Protein	Fat	Carb	Kcal
VEGETABLE (cont'd)	CATS	Tomato Catsup	100	2.00	0.67	25.33	115
	CAUL	Cauliflower—C (Grp B)	100	2.00	0.20	5.00	30
	CELE	Celery—R or C (Grp A)	100	0.75	0.25	3.75	20
	CHIVE	Chives—R	100	3.33	0.00	3.33	27
	CORN	Corn, Yellow	100	3.29	1.34	25.12	126
	CUCU	Cucumber—R (Grp A)	100	0.58	0.20	2.90	16
	EGGPL	Eggplant—C (Grp A)	100	1.22	0.00	6.34	30
	ENDIV	Endive	100	1.20	0.40	3.20	21
	KALE	Kale—C (Grp B)	100	1.85	0.46	5.69	34
	LETT	Lettuce, Iceberg (Grp A)	100	1.00	0.00	2.00	12
	MUSH1	Mushrooms—R	100	2.00	0.57	4.57	31
	MUSH2	Mushrooms, Canned	100	1.92	0.26	5.00	30
	MUST	Mustard Greens—C	100	2.29	0.29	2.14	20
	OKRA	Okra—C (Grp B)	100	1.88	0.13	7.25	40
	ONION	Onions, Raw	100	1.13	0.25	7.38	36
	PARSL	Parsley—R	100	2.33	0.33	7.00	40
	PEAS	Green Peas—R	100	5.38	0.38	14.49	83
	PEPP	Green Peppers—R or C (Grp A)	100	0.80	0.40	5.40	28
	PICK	Dill Pickle Slices	100	0.80	0.00	2.30	12
	POTA1	Potato—Boiled w/o Skin	100	1.70	0.07	20.00	87
	POTA2	Potato—Baked w/Skin	100	2.33	0.10	25.25	111
	RADI	Radish—R (Grp A)	100	0.67	0.44	3.56	21
	SAUER	Sauerkraut—C (Grp A)	100	0.93	0.17	4.32	23
	SPIN1	Spinach—R	100	2.86	0.36	3.57	29
	SPIN2	Spinach, Frozen, w/Butter, Pillsbury	100	3.00	1.00	4.40	39
	SPROU	Bean Sprouts, Mung—R	100	3.08	0.19	5.96	38
	SQUAS	Spaghetti Squash	100	0.64	0.26	6.41	31

Category	Code	Description	Grams	Protein	Fat	Carb	Kcal
VEGETABLE	TOMA	Tomato, Red—R	100	0.89	0.24	4.31	23
(cont'd)	TOMAC	Tomato, Canned in Puree	100	0.84	0.84	5.04	31
	TOMAP	Tomato Paste, Canned	100	3.82	0.92	18.85	99
	TOMPU	Tomato Puree	100	1.68	0.12	10.04	48
	TOMSA	Prego, Spaghetti Sauce w/Meat	100	2.12	5.13	17.88	126
	TURNI	Turnips, Boiled	100	0.77	0.13	4.87	24
	ZUCCH	Zucchini—C (Grp A)	100	1.23	0.15	2.92	18

INDEX

Note: Italic *t* indicates a table on that page. Italic *f* indicates an illustration figure on that page.

Meal planning *(cont'd)*
  calculation examples, 140–142
  caloric calculations in, 13, 25–29, 36,
    54, 73, 77, 76–79, 85, 93–94, 106,
    119–128, 131, 132, 138–139, 188
  carbohydrate/fat/protein ratios in,
    27, 36, 54, 76, 79, 88, 90–91, 94,
    98, 110–115, 122–132, 122t,
    144–146, 154
  carbohydrates, hidden in foods, 64
  chocolate in, 63, 99, 138, 154, 157
  computerized meal planning
    programs, 73, 85–86, 133–134
  creativity in, 105–106, 156
  cross-multiplication and food lists
    in, 135
  desserts and snacks in, , 14, 24, 26,
    73, 81, 85, 86, 90, 162, 166–167
  dietary units in, 129
  emergency meals and, 177
  exchange lists in, 157–158, 182
  extracts and flavorings in, 32, 63,
    105, 154
  fat ratios (*See also* Carbohydrate/fat/
    protein ratio) in, 10–11, 22–23,
    45, 47, 85, 88, 89t, 129–130, 134,
    138, 139, 156, 157, 175, 177
  fine-tuning the diet and, 6–7, 13–14,
    26, 54, 70–95
  flavorings, 32, 63, 105, 154
  food groups in, 12–13, 87
  foods for diet, 62–64
  "free foods" in, 76, 84, 86–87, 154
  fruits, 12, 28, 32, 47, 74, 81, 87, 99,
    104, 106, 134, 154
  gelatin desserts in, 12, 63, 86, 99,
    103, 104, 173–174
  hand calculation of diet and, 133,
    135–137
  illness and, 25–26, 30, 73, 74, 76,
    100–101
  labels, reading ingredient labels for,
    64, 107, 108
  liquid diets (*See* Liquid formula and
    tube feeding)
  measuring (*See* Portion control)
  meats in, 12, 27, 28, 33, 85, 87–88,
    97, 99, 103, 104, 134, 154, 156, 157

medium-chain triglyceride (MCT)
    oil in, 32, 47–49, 84, 88, 101
  nonstick sprays and, 63, 176
  Nutrasweet linked to seizures and,
    90
  nutritional completeness in, 27, 188
  portion control in, 13, 26, 28–29,
    54, 59, 60, 73, 76, 81, 85, 93, 157
  preparing meals in advance in, 97,
    103–104, 155
  processed foods in, 73, 76, 85, 87,
    106–107, 155
  protein ratio (*See also*
    Carbohydrate/fat/protein ratio) in,
    22, 23, 121–123, 122t, 130
  ratios of fat/protein/carbohydrate
    (*See* Carbohydrate/fat/protein
    ratio)
  recipes for, 153–182
  Recommended Daily Allowance
    (RDA) in, 120, 127
  restaurant meals and, 28, 98–100,
    155
  saccharine, 63
  sample plans for, 153–182
  school meals and, 27–28, 98–100
  simple meal example, 176
  snacks (*See* Desserts and snacks)
  sodas in, 63, 81, 83, 90, 100, 155
  soft diets and, 145
  specific foods in, 86–87
  sugar-free vs. carbohydrate-free
    foods in, 64
  sweeteners in, 63, 90, 105
  timesaving tips for, 96–97
  timing/distribution of meals, 76, 81,
    89–90, 130, 139
  travel and vacations and, 28,
    98–100, 104
  variation in, 155
  vegetables in, 12, 28, 31, 32, 47, 74,
    81, 84, 85, 87, 97, 99, 103, 104,
    106, 134, 138, 154, 156, 157
  vitamin/mineral supplements and,
    27, 66, 127, 131, 159, 188
  water/fluid allotment in, 13, 44, 76,
    81–83, 85, 93, 101, 106, 123–124,
    127, 131